NURS
SECRET WAR

Maggie Campbell grew up in Manchester at a time when the city was still on its knees, post-war. She can just about remember the end of rationing! After decades of working as a seamstress in factories, once her children had grown up, Margaret retrained to be a midwife – a career she adored. She now lives in a cottage that overlooks the rolling Pennines where she writes, grows rare dahlias and keeps chickens.

NURSE KITTY'S
SECRET WAR

Maggie Campbell

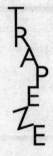

First published in Great Britain in 2020 by Trapeze
an imprint of The Orion Publishing Group Ltd
Carmelite House, 50 Victoria Embankment
London EC4Y 0DZ

An Hachette UK Company

1 3 5 7 9 10 8 6 4 2

A CIP catalogue record for this book is
available from the British Library.

ISBN (Mass Market Paperback) 978 1 4091 9177 3
ISBN (eBook) 978 1 4091 9178 0

Typeset by Born Group
Printed and bound in Great Britain by Clays Ltd, Elcograf S.p.A.

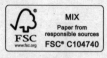

MIX
Paper from
responsible sources
FSC® C104740
www.fsc.org

www.orionbooks.co.uk

For my mother, an avid reader of historical sagas.

Though you're gone, you're still with me in every daft turn of phrase, every old recipe I stumble across and so much of the advice I pass onto my children. Kitty's for you, dear Mum.

PART I

—

1945

Chapter 1

The young American soldier grimaced as he tried to stretch his freshly bandaged arm towards Kitty.

'Please, nurse,' he said, 'stay with me a while longer and read to me. Like you did the other night when I couldn't sleep for the pain.' Beads of sweat ran down the lad's cheeks and onto his clean pyjamas. Yet again, his hair was starting to stick to his ghostly pale forehead.

Kitty shook her head and drew back the curtain around his iron bed. 'Now, just you rest that arm, Glen Hudson,' she said, plumping his pillows. She mopped his brow with a fresh, cool cloth. 'You've got a nasty infection and you're still running a very high temperature. If you want to make your nineteenth birthday and ever get back home to . . . where was it?'

'Des Moines, Iowa, ma'am.'

'Right. Yes, that place. Well, you'd better get some rest.' Lowering her voice, she treated him to her kindest smile, smoothing down his bedsheet. 'And mind you keep our little Hemmingway session to yourself. Look how many other soldiers are on this ward. If you let them know I gave you special treatment, they'll all be having me reading out letters from their sweethearts and bedtime stories. Matron will have my guts for garters. Who'll look after you then?'

Her feverish patient nodded. 'I think I love you, Nurse Longthorne.'

'Get away, you rum pig!' Kitty chuckled. 'If I had a tanner for every delirious GI that said that, I'd be a rich woman!'

Though he was only six years younger than she was, he looked like a lost boy, tucked in as he was with crisp sheets. How much he reminded her of her own brother, Ned, when he'd gone off to war, four years earlier. Except that Glen Hudson's family probably knew their son had returned home from the Rhineland, missing a leg and only barely back from the brink of blood poisoning, but now in the good care of Manchester's Park Hospital. Hitler's armies were falling at last. If Glen survived, he would never have to return to active duty. But what exactly did Kitty and her mother know about poor Ned's fate?

She swallowed hard. She was staring at the clipboard full of Glen's notes in a bid to hide the tears that welled in her eyes, when she felt a tug on her apron ties.

'Nurse Longthorne! Have you a moment?'

A stern voice caused Kitty to look round in alarm. She expected to find Matron, scowling at her with giant, watchful eyes through those round tortoiseshell glasses she wore.

'Oh, Nurse Jones!' Kitty said, so relieved to see instead the bright red hair and freckled cheeks of her friend and fellow-nurse, Violet, that she giggled nervously. She clasped her patient's notes to her chest. 'I thought for a minute you were—'

'Never mind that!' Violet dropped her voice to little more than a whisper. She took the clipboard and hooked it onto the end of the young GI's bed, then pulled Kitty out of earshot. 'I've got something to tell you.'

Kitty felt lightheaded. 'What's wrong?'

'Nothing's wrong,' Violet said. 'Far from it! Come to the staffroom, quick! Churchill's about to address the nation on the wireless.'

'But what if Matron or one of the sisters knows we're—?'

Violet grabbed her hand, squeezing hard. Her cheeks flushed pink. 'They're all there. Even James.' She winked. 'Come on!'

James. Just the very mention of Dr James Williams made Kitty's heart lurch inside her chest. Only two weeks ago, she'd felt sure she was about to officially become the surgeon's sweetheart. She – humble Kitty Longthorne from Hulme – had caught the eye of the best-respected young doctor in Park Hospital, after years of worshipping him from afar, delighting in their blossoming friendship and increasing closeness. But though they had been to a matinee at the cinema and for afternoon tea, which had led to a chaste but enjoyable trip to the Lakes, Kitty was still unsure if they were going steady. Their paths had barely crossed since that picnic on the banks of Windermere. Perhaps he'd been too busy. Or maybe he just saw her as a sympathetic ally and nothing more. She hoped not.

Taking a deep breath, she followed Violet into the crowded staffroom. The early May sunshine streamed in through the large windows, catching the billowing yellow smoke from the doctors' cigars in strong beams of light. Every armchair had been dragged towards the large wooden wireless set that took pride of place on a table in the corner. The doctors sat closest, still wearing their white coats over their suits. Of the nursing staff, Matron sat in front, seated stiffly next to Professor Cecil Baird-Murray. The student nurses who had been allowed to leave their charges stood at the back, chattering excitedly, though the ward sisters treated them to disapproving glances.

With a pang of longing, Kitty spotted James right by the wireless, looking as handsome as ever with his perfectly Brylcreemed dark hair. He rubbed his strong jaw, frowning as he listened over the staffroom hubbub to the broadcaster's preamble. When he leaned over and turned the volume up, Kitty could almost taste the intrigue on the air.

'Do pipe down, everyone!' he shouted, holding his hand up to shush the room's occupants. 'It's starting.'

The crackling sound of radio silence filled the room until Big Ben chimed. Kitty could hardly breathe. When the bell was finally still, Winston Churchill's stately voice rang out, telling the nation that the Germans had surrendered.

'The Act of Unconditional Surrender!' Professor Baird-Murray said, slapping the arm of his chair and pointing with his cigar. 'Did you hear that, gentlemen? The Hun has fallen yet again. About bally time!'

Matron glared at him so that he fell immediately silent, allowing Churchill to speak on.

'Today is Victory in Europe Day.'

Everyone in the staffroom cheered. Those who were seated leaped up, clapping in the direction of the radio. Kitty noticed James steal a glance in her direction. There was pure joy in his eyes for that fleeting moment, but she looked away, listening to the cautious words of Churchill.

'Let us not forget for a moment the toil and efforts that lie ahead.'

She clenched her starched white apron inside her fist, dreading what would inevitably come next.

'Japan, with all her treachery and greed, remains unsubdued . . .'

Edging towards the door, Kitty felt tears bite anew at the backs of her eyes. The war was not yet over for Ned and the other soldiers who had left to fight for Hong Kong in 1941. For all the letters she'd written to him since his departure, not a single one had ever seemed to reach him.

*

'Are you going to get dolled up and go out?' Violet asked, slipping out of her sensible nurse's shoes and unpinning her cap from her glowing red hair which tumbled below her shoulders.

Kitty stood in the doorway to her friend's bedroom, weary after a twelve-hour stint on the ward where she'd worn a smile for her jubilant Allied Forces patients, though her own heart secretly ached. Now, the nurses' home thronged with girls who had come off the day shift, exchanging news of street parties that stretched the length and breadth of the country.

'I've no plans,' she said, 'apart from going to see my mam.'

Violet cast her bundled nurse's uniform onto her bed with abandon. She curled her lip and scoffed. 'Your "mam"! Oh, Kitty! You are funny. You're such a simple Trafford girl.' Then, she held a flowered dress against her body. With its cinched-in waist, it was certainly no home-sewn ensemble.

Biting her tongue against the insult, Kitty stood aside to let Violet hang the garment on the door frame.

'Is that dress silk?' she asked. She watched Violet start to draw dark seams with a fine brush up the backs of her pale legs.

Violet blushed and batted her eyelashes. 'It was a gift. I think VE day calls for making an effort, don't you? Especially as I'm off out with the dashing new beau who bought it for me!'

Kitty looked down at her own dowdy skirt and flat shoes, wondering whether she would have captured the heart of Dr James Williams if she'd worn something other than jumble-sale cast-offs in what little free time she had. 'Well, you'll look just like Rita Heyworth,' she said, forcing a smile. 'Who's the boyfriend?'

Tapping her nose, Violet merely grinned. 'Don't wait up.'

Outside, the spring evening sunshine still warmed Manchester. Everywhere she walked, Kitty found streets hung with colourful bunting and filled with rejoicing people. The children who hadn't been evacuated to the countryside ran around excitedly, their mouths smeared with smiles of bright red jam. Even the red-brick terraces that had been lucky enough to dodge the incendiary bombs of the Luftwaffe seemed to glow with joy at the news that the war was finally over.

When she reached the street in Withington where her mother was lodging above the corner shop, Kitty searched among the revellers. She edged past the long line of tables that were laden with now-empty plates and used napkins. The adults were drinking and dancing the hokey-cokey, and Kitty locked eyes with a little blond boy. He sat alone at the table, holding an uneaten sandwich as if it was a prize.

'Want a butty, miss?' the boy asked, holding his sandwich out to her. 'It's corned beef. I've already had five! We had tinned peaches too.'

Kitty ruffled his hair. 'No thanks, lovey. You enjoy it. Have you seen Mrs Longthorne – the lady who lives over the shop?'

The boy shook his head. He held his fingers up in a V for Victory and Kitty followed suit in reply. She was just about to continue on her way, when an older man lurched into her. Shabbily dressed with his collar open and a stained tie hanging loose, he stank of whisky and his eyes seemed glazed.

'Come 'ere, gorgeous. Give us a peck on the cheek.' He leaned in to kiss Kitty.

'Enjoy your party,' Kitty said, pulling away in horror and marching smartly onwards.

By the time she'd reached the end of the long street, she found Ainsworth's corner shop in darkness with the 'Closed' sign hanging in the window. She pushed the door open with a tinkle of the bell, but the place seemed deserted. The shelves, half empty but for some tins of spam, fruit salad and evaporated milk, thanks to rationing, had apparently been left unguarded.

'Mrs Ainsworth!' Kitty called out.

There was no answer.

She lifted the hinged counter and pushed past the curtain that separated the shop from the living accommodation at the back. Finally, she found Mrs Ainsworth snoozing in her flowery chair, wearing a party hat that was hanging from her neatly curled hair.

Kitty crept past her to open the door that concealed the steep stairs. She climbed up in near-darkness only to find that her mother's room was empty. If she wasn't with the revellers outside and she wasn't here, where was she?

Picking up a photograph that was in a frame beside the neatly made single bed, Kitty looked at the faces in the family portrait that had been taken in 1938, just before war had cast its shadow over the Longthorne family. She traced her finger over the stern faces of her mother, her father, Ned and finally the young, hopeful girl that Kitty had once been, full of nursing ambition and dreams of marrying a doctor – the latter seemed to be slipping beyond her reach. Swallowing the lump in her throat, she knew then exactly where her mother had gone.

Kitty picked her way past the bomb sites and wove through raucous street parties, all the way to Hulme. It was almost dark by the time she reached what had once been her old street.

With a sigh of relief, she finally found her mother, sitting on a battered sideboard that had been left to peel and warp in the rain. Too heavy to carry away and not even broken up for firewood in a city that had been burning for far too long, it was the only piece of their old two-up-two-down home that, miraculously, had been left intact. Everything else had been reduced to rubble by the Nazi bombers.

'Mam! I've walked for miles, trying to find you.' She hopped up next to her mother on the sideboard and flung her arms around her. 'Why aren't you celebrating with Mrs Ainsworth?'

Her mother shied away. When she looked at Kitty in the twilight, it was clear from her bloodshot eyes and the sherry fumes on her breath that she was tipsy.

'I was. But then I had to come back here. I wanted to remember how it was before . . . before we lost everything. All that singing and dancing. VE day, indeed! How can *I* join in? What happens when the Ford factory closes because they don't need me to make parts for Lancaster bombers anymore?' She started to cough. Her chest rattled ominously.

'You'll get a job as a machinist, easy.' Kitty shuffled closer to her mother. 'Something's bound to come up.'

Her mother swallowed a sob. 'And what if it doesn't? What if they find out about your dad? Everybody knows Elsie Longthorne's a laughing stock.'

'It's all yesterday's chip-wrappings, Mam.'

'Oh aye, right,' her mother scoffed. Shaking her head, she finally leaned on Kitty's shoulder. 'You don't see it, do you? The war's over for everyone but us Longthornes.'

'Don't be daft, Mam.'

Then her mother opened her eyes and met Kitty's gaze. 'Daft, am I? Listen! The war's only over for us when the Japanese have surrendered, and they haven't given up the ghost yet.' There were tears in her eyes. She coughed twice. 'What if they don't? What if our Ned *never* comes home?'

'He will! "Missing in Action" doesn't mean dead. And I'll find a way to help with money.' Kitty linked arms with her. 'If Hitler's armies couldn't defeat us, peace certainly won't. It'll all work out. You'll see.'

Her mother shook her head violently. 'No. I won't see. You don't understand.'

'What? What's going on, Mam? There's something you're not telling me. Come on! Out with it.'

With a shaking hand, her mother pulled a crumpled piece of paper from the pocket of her coat. Her chest rumbled and rattled as she passed it to Kitty. 'I got this, this morning.'

Chapter 2

Kitty knew that telegrams rarely contained good news. She smoothed the paper out and, with a sinking heart and feeling her lips prickle with fear, she read the fateful message:

> Deeply regret to inform you that Private Ned Longthorne previously reported as missing after Battle of Hong Kong is now reported prisoner of war interned in Japanese camp stop letter follows stop any further information will be communicated to you immediately stop pending receipt of notification no information should be given to the press stop

She bit her lip and exhaled heavily. 'Oh, Mam!' Tears welled quickly and rolled down her cheeks. Reading and rereading the words, she saw her twin brother in her mind's eye as a ten-year-old. Wearing short trousers and clambering over some old wreck with dirty knees, a snotty nose and boots with flapping soles, Ned had always been the polar opposite of his sister. While she had worked hard at school, loving to read and please her teachers, Ned had taken great joy in playing the truant. He'd made easy money by stealing coal from railway sidings and selling it to the neighbours, and he'd made an excellent lookout while the local thieves peddled their black-market goods on street corners. Best of friends and worst of enemies, depending on which day you caught them on, Kitty and Ned had always been so similar, and yet so very different.

'Our Ned's a prisoner of war?'

'In Japan. Dear God! The Japanese treat them brutal, I've heard.'

'We don't know that for sure. Nobody does. It's all just rumours.'

But her mother's bloodshot eyes were suddenly heavy with more than just sherry. 'Aye. Because the lads never make it back to tell the tale. I feel it in my water. My Ned's suffering out there and he's never coming home.'

Kitty swallowed hard, trying to push away imaginings of her brother, labouring on the Siam-Burma railway or else languishing in some disease-ridden hut in a camp. It wouldn't do to frighten her mother when, in reality, the British public knew so little of what was going on over there. 'You know our Ned, Mam. He's an alley cat with nine lives. Come Christmas Day, we'll all be sitting round the table together, listening to Ned boast about his adventures in the Orient.'

'I haven't got a table anymore. What am I going to buy a new one with? I'm going to be out of collar. You're earning tuppence-ha'penny and need every penny to get you through your training. And as for being together . . . your dad's a dead-leg. And our Ned—' Her body stiffened. She closed her eyes, her mouth downturned. 'I've got the princely sum of nowt.' Her mother jumped down off the sideboard, hands stuffed into her cardigan pockets. She started to walk briskly away.

Jumping down and catching her up, Kitty felt all the joy of VE day draining from her. 'But you've got to hope, Mam. Hope's all we've got left.'

Once her heartbroken, slightly tipsy mother had been safely installed back in her little bedsit, Kitty returned to the nurses' accommodation, treading softly in the newly minted moonlight. She tried the door handle to the block. It was locked.

'What time do you call this?' a voice thundered behind her.

Kitty turned around to see the stern face of Matron, looking formidable in the long shadows with her starched cap perched on top of her perfect battleship-grey curls. She felt the blood drain from her lips, causing her to stumble over her words of explanation. 'I, er – well, it took me hours to walk from – I was visiting my mam, matron. And there were street-parties everywhere. She was crying and we just found out my brother, Ned—'

'It's five past ten, young lady,' Matron said, meaty arms folded over her ample bosom. 'Doors locked and lights out at ten!'

'But—'

'But nothing. Just because it's VE day doesn't mean you can flout the rules. We've just had scores of badly wounded soldiers from the front come in on the trains at Victoria. They're not going to be interested in your excuses if you're not fresh for your shift in the morning.'

'I'm sorry, matron. It won't happen again.' Kitty's words were almost inaudible above the sound of the blood rushing in her ears. She wiped her hands on her skirt. Would her wages be docked as they had been the previous week, when she'd broken that thermometer? How had Matron known to lie in wait for her? Surely she couldn't be the only young nurse who had missed the curfew, tonight of all nights.

'Get inside, then, thoughtless girl!'

Amid her flurry of apologetic words, Kitty was ushered into the utilitarian foyer. The door clanged to behind her and she was left to stumble in the dim light to her room.

Mulling over all that had happened over the last few hours, Kitty sat on her hard bed and slipped her low-heeled shoes off her aching feet. As she rubbed her soles, she tried to imagine what Ned might have gone through after being captured. Her nursing work had been so all-encompassing and the sights in the hospital so grisly on such a regular basis that she'd had to block as many of her true feelings out as possible, just to survive the war. So many young, wounded men whose bodies had been ruined by gunfire and shrapnel! Whenever she and the rest of the medical staff had been unable to save the life of a soldier, she'd fleetingly visualised Ned, lying with a sheet over his face. She'd made an effort to banish such dreadful thoughts as quickly as possible, though.

'Oh, Ned!' she whispered to the shadows cast by her bedside lamp.

Leaning across the rough blankets of her precisely made bed, she lifted the precious framed photograph of her family from its place of honour on the bedside cabinet. Having been shoved by her mother into a drawer of the sturdy old sideboard when her father had been flung into prison, this was one of only two family photographs Kitty had managed to salvage from the wreckage of their bombed-out house. The photograph had been taken at the wedding reception of her cousin, Doreen – a lively affair above The White Lion in Withington in 1938. Doreen and her husband Stanley had both been killed during the Blitz, but here was a snapshot of the Longthornes from better times. Kitty's mother and father were posing in their Sunday best, looking dour. A smiling young Kitty had worn a home-sewn flowery hand-me-down from Maggie, the seamstress who'd lived next door to their terraced house in Hulme. At her father's side stood Ned, drowning in a borrowed suit and grinning from ear to ear. Always smiling. Always a mischievous twinkle in his eye.

'Be careful, our kid,' Kitty said, tracing a finger gently over the face of her twin. 'Mam needs you back in one piece. It would kill her if—'

There was an insistent rat-a-tat knock on Kitty's door, making her jump and drop the frame onto her bed. Who on earth could be paying her a visit after lights out?

Holding her breath, she stood behind the door, poised to open it. 'Hello. Who's there?'

'Open the door this minute, Longthorne!' It was Matron and she sounded even more angry than before.

Gingerly, Kitty opened the door and peered out at the furious face of her superior. Matron's jowls wobbled with indignation.

'You're in trouble, young lady. And not for the first time tonight.'

'Whatever's the matter?' Kitty said, pulling her cardigan tightly around her.

'You've a visitor. A *male* visitor.'

'Eh? Who?'

'Follow me.'

Trotting down the stairs after Matron, listening to the stout woman complain about a male intruder – apparently drunk and disorderly – who had broken a window in the laundry and who had clambered inside the nurses' accommodation block, Kitty could barely stay her wildly beating heart. Who could the man be? It certainly wasn't Ned. And since James's ardour for her had suddenly cooled, it absolutely wouldn't be him.

'Are you sure this gentleman asked to see me?' Kitty asked, spotting her friend Violet slip silently in through the kitchenette window after a night of celebrating.

'He's no gentleman,' Matron said, marching ahead.

A tousled-haired Violet met Kitty's gaze. Wide-eyed, Violet pressed her index finger to her lipstick-smudged lips; begging for Kitty's discretion as she tiptoed past the two, heading in bare feet up the stairs to the bedrooms, holding her high-heeled shoes.

Kitty, however, was more interested to know what man had pursued her to her front door. Matron led her to a storeroom where the caretaker stashed his various tools of the job. She took a key from the large keyring attached to her belt and unlocked the door. Pushing it open, she shed light on the intruder who had been sitting in the pitch-black on a rickety wooden chair.

'Explain!'

The man inside the cupboard held his hand up to squinting eyes and smiled at Kitty with five rotten teeth studded along otherwise toothless gums. 'Hello, love.'

His alcoholic breath billowed out to greet her. Kitty dug her nails into the palms of her hands until the pain made her eyes water. She was almost rendered speechless by the sight of her visitor. Almost.

'*Dad?*'

Chapter 3

'Kitty, love,' her father said. 'Give us a hug.' He was slurring his words, reaching out to her with dirt-ingrained hands.

'What on earth are you doing here, Dad? I thought you were—'

'I got out. Today! A year off my sentence for good behaviour.' He chuckled and winked at the matron. 'I'm a good boy, me!' Then he turned back to Kitty, treating her to a black-toothed smile. 'Your dad's home, Kitty. I've done my time and I'm here to stay.' He almost overbalanced on the chair, righting himself just in time and hiccupping.

Balling her fists, Kitty remembered the sight of her weeping mother, who had had to fend for the family during the war, thanks to her father's thieving ways. 'Well, you're not staying here. You've got no business coming to find me in the middle of the night.'

'I couldn't find your mam. So, I had to find my little girl, didn't I? *She* didn't want to let me in, did you, you fat old cow?' He pointed to Matron, who looked distinctly unimpressed. 'I told her I'm your dad and she didn't believe me. But you can't come between a dad and his girl. And you're all grown-up now, aren't you? My little Kitty-cat's a woman, now.'

Feeling her cheeks flush hot that the matron should be privy to this embarrassing and unexpected reunion, Kitty took a step back. 'I was a woman before you went away.

But you were too busy getting up to no good to notice.' She couldn't disguise the disdain in her voice. Worse still, she couldn't hide the angry tears that stabbed at her eyes. She needed to hold the wave of frustration back. It wouldn't do to make a fool of herself in front of Matron.

'Are you quite all right?' Matron asked her, uncharacteristically placing a hand gently on her forearm. Her formidable superior then faced Kitty's father and treated him to the same stern expression that caused the junior nurses' hearts to quail. 'Perhaps you need to make an appointment, Mr Longthorne. It seems your daughter doesn't want to speak to you right now, and it's a very unseemly late hour.'

'What's it got to do with you, nosey hole?' he said. His face had crumpled into a sneer.

Kitty gasped. 'Dad!'

Unperturbed, Matron took a step towards him, towering over him. 'Out! Out now, or I shall telephone the police.'

As Kitty's father stood up, swaying, then staggered towards them, stinking of unwashed body, stale clothes and alcohol, Kitty backed into the hall. She pressed her hand to her mouth, dreading the consequences of being found to have a degenerate convict for a father. But she could only stand in horror and watch the dreadful spectacle of her father, weaving his way to the door, threatening the matron with all sorts of unpleasantness.

'I'll find out where you live, you fat heifer . . .' he slurred, bouncing off the wall as he staggered outside. 'And I'm going to do your house over.'

Matron, however, was having none of it. 'Be off with you!' She marched after him, chasing him away from the nurses' home. 'And don't come back, or I'll have you arrested, you drunk!'

When he was out of sight, Kitty finally allowed her tears to fall in earnest. She was awash with mixed feelings: shock at having found her supposedly locked-up father, sitting in the caretaker's storeroom; fear of what Matron would think of her and whether his turning up would jeopardise her job; guilt at seeing him shooed away with a flea in his ear like the common criminal he was. The small girl that still dwelled within Kitty, though, had fleetingly been overjoyed to see him, sitting there. She'd almost thrown her arms around him until the stench of beer and whisky had jolted her back into 1945, dispelling her childhood nostalgia like a gust of icy wind blowing away a bad odour.

'Deary me!' Matron said, locking the door and shaking her head. 'What a to-do!' She turned to Kitty and smiled, though it looked as though she was working muscles that didn't often get used. 'Come with me to my office please.'

Swallowing hard, Kitty followed her. She glanced upwards as they passed the staircase but she was so anxious about what Matron might say to her, that she didn't notice her friend Violet, almost entirely concealed behind a wall, peering down at them.

In the Matron's incredibly neat and utilitarian office, Kitty was asked to sit. With a thudding heart, she perched on the edge of an uncomfortable old winged armchair by the fireplace, feeling the springs digging into her bottom. Was she going to get a dressing down? She eyed Matron, who was facing the wall, seemingly busy about something on a small side table. Kitty couldn't see past the woman's broad back and ample behind. What on earth was she doing?

Matron turned round, bearing small glasses of dark liquid. She was wearing that stiff smile again. 'Here. Get this down you, girl. I can see you're all of a two-and-eight. After a shock like that, you look like you could use a sherry. I know I could.'

Kitty accepted the drink and sipped it reluctantly, feeling that at any minute, the Matron would transform back into her usual battle-axe self and berate her for drinking. She wrinkled her nose at the smell. It reminded her too much of her father.

The seat pad of a chintz armchair creaked beneath the weight of the Matron as she took a seat opposite Kitty. 'Now. I need to know I can trust my young nurses, Longthorne, and I don't think you've been entirely honest with me, have you?' She set her sherry glass down on the aspidistra stand by her chair with precision. Her hooded eyes were fixed on Kitty.

Looking down at the small sherry glass, wishing she were anywhere but in this office, Kitty sighed deeply. 'My father's been inside – I mean, in prison for the last two years. He should have served three.' She could hear her own voice starting to crack with grief and humiliation. There was no point in hiding the truth now. 'He was caught stealing silk from the Dunlop balloon factory where my mother worked.'

Matron inhaled sharply. 'I see. Yes. I seem to remember reading about that in the newspaper. It wasn't just an opportunist theft of a single bale, was it?'

Kitty shook her head and bit her lip. She couldn't look up to face the hawk-eyed scrutiny of the matron. 'It was a big robbery. Quite big. I mean—'

'Several large trucks full of silk, I heard.' Matron pursed her lips. 'Didn't that robbery scupper the manufacture of barrage balloons for weeks?'

There was no way Kitty could keep the hot blotches from itching their way up her neck, spreading to cover her cheeks in a vivid shade of mortified red. She shrugged. *Come on, Kitty! Now's not the time to get tight-lipped!* She needed to win Matron's heart – *if* she had one. 'It's been a nightmare for me and my mam, if I'm honest,' she began. 'Mam was working as a machinist at Dunlop, so they gave her her marching orders when my dad got collared for the robbery. She didn't know a thing about it until the coppers turned up at our door. I swear. Look, I'm sorry I didn't say anything when I started working here, but . . . the other nurses are all from such good families, and I thought if you knew—'

'If I knew your father was a convicted thief?'

Kitty nodded. 'My mam has had to work so hard to keep us going during the war. Our Ned's . . . I found out today that my twin brother's a prisoner of war in a Japanese camp. Maybe he'll never come home. There's just me and Mam, really. She wanted better for me than what she had. And she always says, "Lie with dogs, Kitty Longthorne, and you'll get fleas." So, what I'm saying is, neither of us care to have anything to do with my dad. He's bad news. We know that. Please don't sack me, matron.'

With a grunt, Matron stood and smoothed her starched uniform down. 'It's our little secret. You can't choose your relatives. I realise that. But you'll have to work doubly hard to earn my trust and respect, young lady, now that I know you've been keeping such a scandal from me. I'll be watching you.' Her face had hardened again and she was now the matron all the nurses feared and revered. 'Off to bed with you and we will not mention this again.'

'Yes, matron. Thanks, matron.' Looking down at her slippers, Kitty half-curtsied and scurried out of the office and back up to her room as fast as she could.

*

As she lay in her hard bed, staring at the shadows that played on the ceiling, she thought about how this should have been the best of days. Hitler had surrendered. The whole of Manchester had been celebrating. Hope hung heady on the summer air.

She rummaged in the little drawer of her bedside cabinet and felt for the prized postcard that James had sent her a full year earlier, when he had attended a surgeon's conference in Chicago. Putting on her lamp, she traced a finger over the photograph of the city skyline and then turned the card over to reread his tiny, tight handwriting.

> *My Dearest Kitty,*
> *Chicago is indeed the windy city – all the bleaker for you not being here. The scale of the place! I saw the sun rise over Lake Michigan this morning. Spectacular! But it didn't warm my day as much as your smile. After the war, we'll visit together.*
> *Yours, as ever,*
> *James*

She kissed his signature and propped the postcard against the lamp base. By rights, VE day should have heralded the dawn of a bright new era in the story of Kitty Longthorne – the promise of a future with the doctor she loved, doing a job she adored in peacetime. Yet, the reappearance of her father on the scene threatened to sour everything. She was lucky that Matron had been so forgiving. Nursing was a profession where reputation mattered, and Bert Longthorne was a convicted criminal. Her mother had only just begun to rebuild a life for herself, and Bert Longthorne was bad news for any woman foolish enough to let him get close. Kitty *had* to keep the infernal dead-leg out of her affairs and away from her mother.

Do I tell Mam or keep it to myself? she wondered. *Will Dad be able to find Mam if I keep quiet about where she's lodging?*

The last thing Kitty thought about before she fell into a troubled sleep was that, as long as Matron kept her confidence, things might turn out fine. Nobody else knew the sordid secrets of the Longthorne family.

Did they?

Chapter 4

'Just keep your arm as relaxed and still as you can!' Kitty told Glen, who was staring down at the syringe in her hand. He was wearing a look of pure horror, a thermometer poking out of his grimacing mouth.

Though her patience was frayed after a sleepless night, worrying about her father's visit, her mother's safety and how the matron's discovery of her lie might affect her future, she gently took his arm. 'Look away, cocker. You'll hardly feel it.'

Her patient shook her loose and spat the thermometer onto the bedclothes. 'Wait! No! I-I can't,' he said.

Kitty tutted. 'Can't what? Come on, Glen Hudson! After everything you told me about the carnage you've lived through . . . And you're letting a tiny little needle bother you?'

He tried to wriggle away from her, clutching the bedsheets tightly to his chest. 'It hurts like stink, that stuff.'

'More than having your leg blown to smithereens by a mine?'

He nodded, sweating furiously, though she knew the sheen on his face was down to his spiking temperature, rather than fear. His breath smelled sickly above the sharp tang of disinfectant that pervaded the ward. Kitty's fellow junior nurse, Lily Schwartz, was mopping her way along the ward towards them. She smiled sympathetically at her colleague, who was enduring the usual cat-calling from a delirious German prisoner of war, three beds away. Kitty didn't know if it was better or worse that Lily could understand everything the Nazi captive was saying. By rights, he should have been on another ward, with the other prisoners of war, but a recent influx of wounded German soldiers had their dedicated, high-security ward busting at the seams. Sadly, Kitty reflected, the military police officer who sat by his bed never told his German charge to pipe down.

'Look, I know it's not nice,' she said, turning her attention back to Glen and the oily mixture in the syringe. 'But you need penicillin if you're going to get better.' She considered her mother who coughed and coughed, thanks to the chronic bad chest that had come from years of her working in factories and living in damp houses. Except, like so many working-class civilians, who suffered in dirty, dangerous workplaces or who had been caught up in the Blitz and left to rot in whatever temporary shelter they could find, her mother couldn't afford to see a specialist. 'Just think yourself lucky. If you weren't in the military, there's no way you'd get these new antibiotics, and you could wave goodbye to what's left of your leg . . .' She eyed the bandaged stump, where his leg had been removed below the knee. 'If not your life!'

Her patient was so reluctant that Kitty had to call on Lily for support. 'Give us a hand, will you? Glen, here, is giving me a run for my money.' She tried her best to conceal her impatience from the young soldier. Though her shift didn't end for many hours, the need to escape the hospital and warn her mother that her jailbird father was on the prowl felt more urgent than ever.

'No! No!' Glen cried. 'Why are you doing this to me, nurse?'

Lily abandoned her mop and bucket to hold the young American down. Though she was tiny in build, her grip was iron. 'Hush, Glen! You know Nurse Longthorne is only trying to help you,' she said.

Glen was so distracted by Lily's German accent that he held still long enough to be jabbed. He called out in pain as the thick medicine was delivered into his bloodstream. When Kitty had first started to be trusted with administering the penicillin intravenously and with needles generally, she'd winced every time she punctured a soldier's skin. Watching people suffer and die had been the part of her job that had taken the most getting used to, but after a while, she had hardened to the idea of causing a patient pain. And today, Kitty was preoccupied by family matters.

'You're a Nazi spy!' Glen said to Lily, clutching ruefully at his arm. He was speaking too fast. His eyes were wide and staring. The fever had got a hold of him. 'Like that Kraut prisoner of war down the way.'

Lily smiled at him kindly. If she was hurt by his harsh accusation, she didn't show it. 'I've lived here since I was twelve. I'm no more a Nazi spy than you.' She spoke softly, patting the soldier's good shoulder, though he shrank from her touch. 'And the war's over.'

The door to the ward slammed open and Sister Iris loomed in the doorway. 'Nurse Schwartz! What are you doing to that poor young man?'

Kitty watched her companion pale at the sight of the stern sister. How Kitty wanted to put herself between their towering superior – made even more formidable by her starched cap and horn-rimmed glasses – and the tiny Lily.

She knew, however, that any attempt at heroism would be futile. It always was. Sister Iris's fists were balled. Her cheeks were flame-red. Nothing could stand in the path she was beating to Lily.

'I-I was just helping Longthorne, sister. I was talking to the patient to calm him.' Lily's lips trembled as she spoke.

'She's a spy!' the delirious young American added unhelpfully.

Further down the ward, the German prisoner of war, whose entire upper body was bandaged, thanks to burn injuries, shouted something that Kitty didn't understand, though his mocking tone of voice was clear enough. Suddenly, she felt like she and Lily were in a market square, being jeered at by an angry mob and pelted with rotten vegetables for consorting with the enemy.

'Nurse Schwartz was just helping me administer the antibiotics, sister,' she said. 'Honest. It needed two of us. Young Glen, here, is near hallucinating with his fever.'

'Silence, Longthorne, or I'll have you disciplined for insubordination!' Sister Iris yelled, glaring at Kitty whilst grabbing little Lily by the upper arm and yanking her back towards the mop and bucket. She focused her ferocity back onto Lily. 'Get on with your cleaning, girl!'

Perhaps because he didn't understand what was being said, the German prisoner of war continued to call out to Lily.

Sister Iris turned to him, almost melting him with a look of pure volcanic fury. She wrenched his bedraggled bedclothes over his legs and tucked them in so tightly that he whimpered and then fell quiet. 'And *you*! Just be glad that you're being treated and lying in a clean British hospital bed, which is more than I can say for our own lads caught behind Jerry enemy lines.' She glared at the military policeman sitting by his bedside, daring him to chip in with an unwanted smart alec remark, but he was silent.

Kitty's heart beat wildly as she collected the used syringe and soiled dressings from her patient's nightstand. The war in Europe was over, but in Park Hospital, a battle still raged on between the junior and senior staff. Surely Sister Iris would continue her rounds, now that she'd reminded everyone who was in charge.

When Sister Iris locked eyes with Kitty, however, and beckoned her over to where she was now standing at the foot of a newly empty bed, Kitty knew something was amiss. She swallowed hard.

'Yes, sister?'

Iris sneered down at her through those horn-rimmed glasses. 'You're quite the talking point in the staffroom today, Nurse Longthorne.'

Keeping as still as she possibly could, Kitty willed herself to appear unruffled. Had Matron betrayed her confidence? 'Oh?'

The tall sister leaned in. 'Let's just say news travels fast on the grapevine. I'll be keeping my eye on you.'

'I-I don't know what you mean,' Kitty said, fighting tears of frustration and shame that her family secret was almost certainly out. Was this the beginning of the end of her dreams of a nursing career? Worse still, could James have been privy to whatever tittle-tattle had gone on in the staffroom?

'Oh, come now. Don't try that "butter-wouldn't-melt" act with me, young lady. I've got your ticket.' Wearing the glimmer of a nasty smile, Sister Iris seemed satisfied that she'd set the cat among the pigeons enough to ruffle everyone's feathers. On flat feet in her sensible lace-up shoes, she marched out of the ward, leaving the door to slam behind her.

'Are you all right, Lily?' Kitty whispered, putting her arm round her colleague who was crying silently as she mopped under a bed.

Lily looked at her with reddened eyes and smiled weakly. 'Are you?'

'We can't let her grind us down. It's what she wants. She's just toying with us for sport.' Kitty swallowed hard. She was putting on a brave face for Lily but inside, she was quaking with fear and anger. Should she confront Matron about the apparent gossip? What exactly had been said? Perhaps she should talk to James about the sister's pointed comments. Yes. He was wise and said he cared about her.

Finishing her duties on the ward was agony. Ideally, she needed to get to her mother at the Ford factory in Trafford, though she knew it was impossible until her shift was over. Every bang or clatter had Kitty looking at the door to the ward, expecting either Matron or her stinking drunk of a father to appear at any moment.

As soon as she'd changed the dressings on the last patient, she hastened down towards the operating theatre, where she knew she'd find the surgeon of her dreams.

Peering through the glass panes of the doors, she spotted her friend Violet. Despite her late night of apparent revelry, Violet was looking fresh-faced and positively glowing. She stood next to a patient who, with his severely injured face exposed, looked prepped for delicate facial surgery. With a pang of jealousy, she watched as Violet passed one of her long, silken hairs to the surgeon who was instantly recognisable as Kitty's sweetheart, James. Even beneath his utilitarian scrubs, James looked dashing and devilishly handsome.

Kitty watched with mixed feelings as he threaded his needle with Violet's sterilised hair – the secret weapon of Manchester's most acclaimed prodigy in the emerging field of plastic surgery. The staff of Park Hospital cooed over how their very own Dr James Williams had had the bright idea of using hair instead of the usual surgical thread to stitch facial wounds and thereby lessen scarring, and, of course, only Violet's hair had been long and strong yet fine enough to do the job. Everybody complimented Violet on the medicinal use of her silken tresses.

Kitty touched her own decidedly ordinary mousy hair and felt dowdy beyond belief at that moment. As she watched Violet assist James and noticed how their eyes smiled as they looked at one another, Kitty felt a lump of sadness lodge in her throat. Did he look at her that way? She couldn't be sure.

In the background, the hospital's new anaesthetist, Richard Collins, stood by, looking quite the gooseberry. Clearly, Kitty wasn't the only person who had picked up on the chemistry between James and Violet – or was it merely Kitty's overheated imagination? James said something to Violet and she giggled coquettishly in response. That much was evident, even though they both wore surgical masks.

It was only when her short fingernails started to dig into her palms and sting that Kitty realised she'd been clenching her fists hard. *Pack it in, Kitty,* she counselled herself, *you're being daft.* She exhaled deeply and imagined locking her blossoming jealousy and hurt in a box.

When the surgery was over and the sleeping patient wheeled away, Kitty knocked timidly on the operating theatre doors.

'Dr Williams! Can I have a moment, please?' She could hear the tremor in her own voice and silently castigated herself for being so apologetic.

James was scrubbing his arms and hands at the sink. He looked over to her but there was no smile playing around his eyes now. His puzzled expression quickly transformed into a solemn grimace. 'Nurse Longthorne.' He hesitated, clearly considering his words.

Violet busied herself with collecting the bloodied surgical instruments, turning her back on her friend. It was almost as if someone had opened a window or another door in the theatre, allowing an icy wind to gust through. Only Richard Collins treated Kitty to a merry wave and a warm smile.

'I needed to ask you something of a personal nature,' Kitty said to James, hopefully. 'And it can't really wait.'

Glancing over at Violet, James cleared his throat and raised an eyebrow. 'I'm sorry, nurse. I hardly think that would be appropriate. I'm terribly busy. I don't have a moment.'

'But—'

'Could you close the door on your way out, please? There's a good girl.'

And just like that, the man she had fallen head over heels for, long before he had ever asked her out, had dismissed her. The shaft of sunlight that their fledgling romance had hitherto cast on her otherwise drab life had been snuffed out by an ominous, dark cloud of notoriety that now hung over Kitty and dogged her every step.

Her dreams were dashed.

Her bright future was over and done with.

Chapter 5

'Ah! Here she is! At last,' Violet said, setting her knife and fork down carefully. Her hearty voice cut through the low-level hubbub in the nurse's dining room. There was no hint of her having witnessed Kitty's devastating rejection by James only an hour or so earlier. 'Here's our Kitty. I saved a place for you.' She slapped the empty chair to her right. 'We were all starting to worry there was something up, weren't we, girls?'

The other junior nurses nodded fervently, all smiles. Had they heard about Kitty's late-night visitor?

'Come on, Kitty, chuck! It's tater hash,' Molly, the tuberculosis nurse from Urmston said. She shovelled a spoon of the grey-looking stew into her mouth, as if demonstrating quite how delicious it was. 'Your favourite.'

All eyes were now on Kitty. Even Matron and the off-duty sisters on the top table were staring her way, commenting out of earshot with their hands covering their mouths. Sister Iris was right. The senior staff, at least, all knew.

Kitty felt her cheeks flush hot. She helped herself to the last of the potato hash, which she could see contained only a measly portion of corned beef, and took her seat next to Violet. Would the others notice her red-rimmed eyes?

'Are you quite all right, Kitty? You look terribly . . . off colour,' Violet said.

It wouldn't do to let even her closest friend know that she'd been crying in the lavatories – certainly not in front of the others. 'I'm absolutely fine,' she said, unfurling her napkin. 'And I'm famished after such a gruelling morning.'

Spooning the now cold stew into her mouth, Kitty stole another glance at the matron. Was it conceivable that such a respected woman could have tittle-tattled in the staffroom to James and the other doctors? Dare she confront her superior over the matter?

No. She needed to get away from this stifling atmosphere. The hospital was *her* prison at that moment, and all Kitty wanted to do was find her mother, warn her about her father's return and cry on her shoulder. True, the patients on the ward needed nursing care, but they had other girls to tend their needs. Her mother, on the other hand, only had Kitty to look out for her, and Kitty wasn't about to shirk her duty to the woman who had sacrificed everything to give her daughter a good start in life.

An idea quickly took shape, though it would take some daring to pull off. 'Actually, I do feel a little peaky,' she said, as breathlessly as she could. 'Ooh, I say!'

Keeling over suddenly, so that she practically knocked the solidly built Molly from her seat, Kitty pretended to faint – or at least swoon, since she knew a room full of qualified and experienced nurses would work out in a jiffy that her blood pressure was fine and that she hadn't lost consciousness at all. She slumped to the floor between the chairs and winced when her head hit the parquet.

'Good Lord! Whatever is the matter?' Matron said, rising quickly from her table and striding over to Kitty. 'Give her room, Molly! Violet, raise her legs!'

Groaning, Kitty opened her eyes to find Matron's ruddy, stern face only inches above hers. With a well-scrubbed hand, Matron patted her sharply on the cheek.

'Longthorne! Longthorne! Are you all right? Look at me, Kitty!'

Kitty made sure that she was a limp, dead weight. There was a flurry of activity and complaint as she was hoisted to her feet. It took matron, Violet and Molly to get her upright and back onto her chair.

'Have some water,' Matron said, thrusting a glass to her mouth. 'Here. Drink! What a to-do!'

'Sorry, matron,' Kitty mumbled, wracking her brains for a convincing story that would get her out of the rest of her shift. Surely, her period would provide a useful excuse. 'I'm unwell.' Yet, the Matron's expression was still unforgiving. 'Or maybe I've caught something off one of the patients.'

Matron's lips thinned to a line. 'If you want to be a sister or even a matron one day, young lady, you're going to have to be more robust than this. Up you get!'

Surely the matron wasn't that hard-hearted!

'Follow me!'

Where was the matron taking her?

Kitty followed her into the corridor where they were out of earshot of the others in the dining room. Matron stopped in the doorway to a store cupboard and lowered her voice. Her eyes softened. 'It's small wonder that you're swooning after all that's gone on, but I don't want the others thinking I'm a soft touch. Get some rest. You can start fresh tomorrow.'

It was the stroke of luck that Kitty needed! 'Thank you, matron. I really appreciate it. I do feel dreadful. But can I ask you one thing?'

'Of course.'

'Does anyone know about my father? Last night, I mean?' She screwed the corner of the apron up into a sweaty ball.

Confronting the woman who was tantamount to a nursing goddess was a daring move, but one she had to make, nevertheless.

Matron raised an eyebrow, blinking hard. 'Do you mean, have I told anyone else?' A shadow seemed to fall over them both and the corridor felt suddenly colder. 'Gossiping? What sort of woman do you take me for?'

'Sorry, matron. It's just Sister Iris said—'

'What Sister Iris said is not my concern. Now, off to bed with you before I have a change of heart.'

Kitty had had a lucky escape, both from her nursing duties and the matron's wrath. In the privacy of her room, she quickly changed her clothes, hanging up her uniform neatly in her small wardrobe and donning a raincoat over her plain skirt and hand-knitted jumper. Leaving her cushions stuffed beneath her bedclothes to make it look like someone was asleep in her bed, she slipped out of the back door of the nurses' home.

Outside, the hopeful spring sunshine had given way to a typical Mancunian downpour. Walking quickly to the bus stop, Kitty was glad of being able to shield her face behind her umbrella. It was essential that her absence went unnoticed by the other staff. If she got caught, she'd almost certainly lose her job.

She was so upset by James's rejection in the operating theatre and preoccupied by her plans to get to the Ford factory that she noticed neither the freezing rain seeping through her shoes, nor the dishevelled man who emerged from behind a tree and followed her. The trolleybus splashed to a halt alongside the kerb and Kitty jumped on the back, greeting the conductress. Could it be that all the conductresses would lose their jobs now that their male counterparts were set to return to Civvy Street? she wondered. Perhaps so, given the woman's glum face, or maybe she was just the worse for wear after a night of VE day celebrations.

Taking her seat further inside, downstairs, where the smell of diesel and wet upholstery was strongest, Kitty stared blankly through the steamed-up windows. The merry ding-ding of the trolleybus's bell as they set off towards Trafford seemed far too jolly, given her personal circumstances.

The conductress walked past her to collect fares from the front of the bus, chit-chatting with the other travellers about their own festivities and what they hoped for the future.

Kitty searched in her purse for the bus fare. She registered the stink of stale beer behind her just before a gravelly voice said, 'Morning, Kitty, love!' right by her ear.

Spinning around with a thudding heart, she caught sight of her father. He was sprawled across an entire double seat. In the cold light of day, he looked even more dirty and destitute.

'I knew I hadn't seen the last of you! That would have been too easy.' She felt the other passengers looking her way. 'What do you want, Dad? I've got nowt to say to you.'

'Oh, don't be like that, our Kitty.' Her father leaned forward, gripping the steel bar of Kitty's seat. 'I've served my time, you know. I've paid my debt. And now, I want to come home to my family, except I can't find your mam.'

And I'm leading him right to her! Kitty mused. *I can't do right for doing wrong.* She glanced at the conductress and the other men on the bus, wondering whether they'd come to her aid if she couldn't shake off her father. The men were all elderly, however. The conductress was no more than five feet tall. No, Kitty was on her own.

'You should have thought of that before you robbed the Dunlop factory,' she said, spitting the harsh words out almost under her breath so that nobody but her father could hear her.

'I was just trying to make ends meet, love.' Her father rubbed the overgrown stubble on his chin. There was regret in his eyes, but that might just be too much hard-living.

'You? You never put food on our table. That was always down to Mam. Anything you earned was for you. Fancy tailored suits and Italian shoes, even though we were freezing and starving. Whatever was left, disappeared in the bookies. So don't talk to me like you're some heroic provider.'

Her father sucked in air sharply through his rotten teeth. 'That's harsh. I just want my wife and children back. I'm ready to turn over a new leaf.'

Kitty could feel the anger fizzing inside her. She paused to pay the conductress her bus fare. Disappointingly, her father had enough change to cover his fare, which he counted out with blackened fingernails. No chance of him being thrown off the bus.

'What do you know about your wife and children?' Kitty whispered. 'Our Ned's languishing in a prisoner-of-war camp in Japan, if you must know.'

Her father's face dropped; his eyes wide with surprise. 'No. You're lying.'

'Am I? A lot's happened while you've been off, enjoying a holiday at Her Majesty's pleasure.' She narrowed her eyes and scrutinised her father. 'You remember he enlisted, don't you?'

'Course I do! I waved him off on the train. It's like it was yesterday.'

'Really? Are you sure about that? Because the way I remember it, you weren't there. It was me and Mam. Mam, crying her eyes out when he left. Mam, crying her eyes out when we got the telegram, saying he was missing in action in the Far East. You should have been the one to go off and fight. Not him.'

Her father examined the scabs on his knuckles and scratched at the mole on his nose. 'I've always had a bad back.'

'Didn't stop you when you were lifting stolen gear off the back of a lorry, though, did it? Why are you really here, Dad? What do you want?' She was wracking her brains as to how she could shake her father off her tail before she reached the Ford factory.

'I've told you. I want to see your mam.' He reached out to touch the collar of her raincoat, but Kitty backed away.

'She doesn't want to see you.'

Shaking his head, looking more hangdog than she thought possible, her father's voice cracked when he spoke. 'I'm sorry you can't believe I'm a changed man, our Kitty. But I shouldn't be surprised. Nobody did ever think much of Bert Longthorne. How can I act like a fine upstanding gentleman when you all treat me like a ne'er do well and a cad?'

Kitty gripped her handbag hard, tempted to box her father's ears with it. But seeing the other passengers stealing glances their way, she opted to maintain her composure. 'Leave us be, Dad. What will it take to convince you? Mam and me – we don't need you in our lives, now. You weren't there when we needed you but we muddled through in spite of you.'

Her father ran his hand through greying, greasy hair and brushed the dandruff off the shoulders of his ragged suit. 'You're hard, like your mother, you are. You might be all fancy-Dan and a nurse, now, but you're made of stone. That's not a Longthorne heart in your chest.'

By now, the terraced housing and bomb sites had slid out of view. They'd ventured into the grimy industrial heart of Trafford, rumbling by factories that belched smoke as though live dragons were tethered inside, smelting the metal with their fiery breath for those Lancaster bombers and tanks and guns. The bus bounced over a pothole, and Kitty realised she was about to miss her stop. Somebody had rung the bell. She'd have to leave it to the last minute to sprint for freedom if she were to avoid her father following her.

As if he read her mind that the conversation was over, her father cleared his throat. 'Lend your old dad a few bob, will you? Just 'til I get some work.'

Ah. There it was. Her father had a price just high enough to get him an afternoon in the pub. Kitty took a few shillings from her purse and threw them into his lap so that they scattered on the floor. The bus had juddered to a halt. Two other passengers had got off and if she didn't hurry, the bus would pull away. The bell ding-dinged.

'Wait your hurry!' she shouted to the conductress. 'I want to get off, here.'

Grabbing her bag and barging her way to the back, she disembarked and sprinted off down the street. When she looked behind her, she couldn't see her father on the bottom deck but nor was he running after her.

'Calm down, Kitty,' she told herself. 'He'll just be scavenging for those coins like the rat he is.'

She hastened down the street and crossed the tram tracks to the Ford factory – acres of industrial warehousing that looked like a veritable maze of brick, glass and steel – wondering how on earth she'd single out her mother from more than seven thousand other women, all manufacturing parts for Lancaster bombers. Kitty wasn't sure of the precise nature of the work that her mother and the other women did, but it sounded like dirty, dangerous and impressive work.

'I'm here to see Elsie Longthorne,' she said to the receptionist in a damp space that smelled of engine oil and metal. 'It's really urgent. Family stuff.' She couldn't help but glance over her shoulder to check that her father wasn't lurking outside in the rain.

The receptionist stared at her glumly and shifted her gaze to a large clock on the wall. 'Her shift doesn't finish for hours.'

'It's an emergency.'

Ten agonising minutes of waiting later and Kitty's mother appeared, wearing overalls that were blackened from grease with her hair tied up in a scarf. She was wiping her hands on a cloth.

'Whatever's the matter, Kitty?' she asked, her brow furrowed. 'Is it our Ned? Have you heard summat?' She started to cough violently, covering her mouth with an oily hand.

Kitty pulled her outside into the rain and covered her with her umbrella. 'I'm sorry, Mam. I had to warn you.'

Her mother coughed again. 'Warn me about what?'

'Dad's been let out. He's trying to find you. I've already sent him packing twice, but—'

Fear, regret, guilt and disgust seemed to cast shadows of varying darkness over her face as she listened, wide-eyed. 'No,' she said. She clutched Kitty's arm, started to cough and shake her head. 'No! No! No! You've got to keep him away from us. Promise me, Kitty. Promise!'

Suddenly, she grabbed at her stomach, coughing and coughing until blood spattered onto her chin – a dazzling shade of red in the pouring rain beneath those grey skies. Her eyes rolled back in her head and she slumped onto Kitty.

'Mam!'

Chapter 6

'Oh Violet. I'm glad you answered. I'm in a terrible pickle,' Kitty told her friend, holding her hand around the mouthpiece of the telephone in a bid to foil the eavesdropping, gossip-hungry receptionist. She stole a glance down at her mother, laid across several seats in the Ford factory reception, clutching at a bloodied white handkerchief. She was deathly pale, though the coughing had now calmed, at least. Kitty reached out to rub her ankle affectionately. 'My mother's really worryingly ill. She needs a doctor urgently. Tell Dr Williams. I don't know who else to turn to.'

'James – I mean, Dr Williams – is in clinic. Can't you get a GP to look her over?' Violet sounded perplexed.

Kitty blushed. 'We can't afford it.'

'Take her to the Royal Infirmary, if she's that bad.'

'She won't go. Look, just tell Dr Williams. I'm sure he'll help.'

'All righty,' Violet said breezily on the other end. 'Give me the address.'

Kitty relayed the address of her mother's bedsit, above Mrs Ainsworth's corner shop in Withington.

There was a pause on the crackling line. Was Violet writing it down? 'Leave it with me,' she said. 'Got to dash!' The line went dead.

Turning to her mother, Kitty treated her to a weak smile. 'I really think we should get you to the hospital, Mam. I've left a message for James, but—'

Her mother clutched at her hand, wheezing as she spoke. 'Just get me home, love. Get me into my bed and make me a nice cuppa. There's a good girl. I'll be right as rain tomorrow.' She started to cough. Her chest rattled ominously but, thankfully, there was no more blood. 'I'm not paying half a crown to see some quack. All I need is a good night's kip.'

Word of Elsie Longthorne's collapse evidently had travelled fast via the switchboard, as one of the directors came down from his office and insisted on taking them both wherever they needed to go in his Wolseley.

Kitty looked out of the window. There was no sign of James, driving down the road in his Ford Anglia. 'If you could run us over to Manchester Royal Infirmary, that would be grand, thanks,' Kitty said, helping her mother to her feet.

But her mother held her hand up. 'No! No hospitals. Take me home. Please.'

The large, gleaming car seemed out of place on the cobbled, terraced street where her mother lodged above the corner shop. Those who weren't at work came out on their front steps to get a better look – women with their hair concealed beneath headscarves, wearing aprons over their clothes and carpet slippers on their feet. Kitty watched them, chatting among themselves, presumably speculating about the circumstances surrounding Mrs Longthorne being helped into the shop by a well-dressed gentleman with a fine car.

'There you go, Elsie,' the manager said, helping Kitty's mother onto her bed. 'I'll leave you in the good care of your daughter, here. But I do suggest you see a doctor. Would you like me to arrange for one to visit you?'

Her mother shook her head violently. 'No, ta. I'm just sickening for something. I'll be back in work tomorrow. I promise, Mr Travis. I'm not shirking.'

He stood to attention and saluted stiffly. 'Right you are, ma'am. Get well soon.'

Once he was gone, Kitty helped her mother to change into her nightgown. She made a fire in the small cast-iron fireplace, heated an enamel bowl full of water and gently cleaned the blood and oil from her mother's hands and face with a clean, soapy rag. 'You're burning up. Come on, Mam. Let's get you into bed.'

With her mother tucked in, she boiled the kettle and brewed a pot of strong tea for them both, spooning jam into her mother's cup to give her some much-needed energy.

'Now, shall I read to you?' Knowing that reading wasn't her mother's strongest suit, Kitty took a pocket romantic novel from her handbag. 'This is as good as any Heddy Lamar film.'

'No, Kitty, love,' her mother said. Her voice was hoarse and rumbling. 'Put the wireless on. Stay with me a while. We'll listen to *Woman's Hour*, eh? And then I'll get some kip.'

They sat in companionable silence, listening to the beautifully enunciated received English voice of the programme's lady presenter, coming from the sunburst-shaped speaker of the wooden wireless that sat on her mother's battered old dressing table. The end of the war was the talking point of the day and the mood at the BBC was jubilant. Kitty, however, could barely concentrate on what was being said. Her mind was in turmoil over how she might get her mother seen by a doctor. If only she'd agreed to be taken to the hospital, she could have received the necessary examination, tests and emergency treatment there. Now, they'd have to find half a crown to see the GP – assuming her mother would even agree to it. Did she have some nasty cancerous growth taking root in her chest? Had she somehow contracted the dreaded tuberculosis? Or was she lucky enough that the coughing had merely caused a blood vessel in her throat to rupture? No. The Longthornes weren't lucky enough for whatever ailed her mother to be benign.

Glancing sideways at her pale-faced patient, Kitty saw that her mother had drifted off to sleep. Squeezing her own eyes shut and exhaling a long and ragged breath of her own, Kitty rose from her chair and softly made her way onto the little landing her mother shared with her landlady. She sat at the top of the dark, steep stairwell and sobbed silently into her hands.

I can't cope, she thought. *It's all too much, what with Ned and Dad and James being a pig. If Mam were to . . .* Even in the privacy of her own thoughts, Kitty couldn't readily countenance her mother dying. And yet, given the dirty industrial work she'd had to take on during the war and the jobs she'd had in factories before as a machinist, sewing raincoats, where the air had been thick with the fumes of waterproof glue and fibres from the cutting table, would it be any wonder if her mam *was* suffering the unthinkable?

The door below opened, suddenly flooding the stairwell with dazzling daylight. Mrs Ainsworth appeared at the foot of the stairs, grunting as she started to climb.

Kitty got to her feet, quickly wiping her eyes.

Mrs Ainsworth looked up, her ugly black hair net almost slipping over her left eye. 'Oh, there you are! How is she?' she whispered.

'She's sleeping,' Kitty said.

The landlady paused midway up the stairs, audibly out of breath. 'Well, you've got a visitor. A gentleman. I can't be doing with gentleman callers, mind. I've got customers to serve out front. Only this one says he's a doctor.'

At the bottom of the stairwell, their mysterious visitor appeared, wearing a fine camel overcoat. He was clutching his brown felt trilby to his chest with one hand and carried a bulging leather doctor's bag in the other. 'Miss Longthorne.'

'Jame— I mean, Dr Williams!' Kitty steadied herself against the wall and backed further onto the landing. Her heart was a fluttering hummingbird inside her chest. 'You came.'

A flicker of a smile warmed his solemn face. 'Of course. I don't know who took down the note and your mother's address, but it was purely by chance one of the trainee nurses happened upon it. It had been abandoned by the telephone. Luckily, my name was at the top. No matter! Now, can I come up and see the patient? Mrs Ainsworth? If you'd be so kind.'

Flustered and giggling, Mrs Ainsworth descended in a flurry of creaking stairs. 'Silly me! Sorry, doctor! Can I make you a nice cuppa?'

Eventually, with a little charm and flattery, James managed to shoo the old fusspot back behind the counter of the shop. Kitty and her doctor were alone.

Wondering if she should mention Violet's betrayal, but deciding it was not the time for tittle-tattle, Kitty helped James out of his overcoat and draped it carefully over the old armchair by the fire. 'I'm so, *so* glad to see you. Thank you.'

He set his doctor's bag down on the end of Kitty's mother's bed and opened it up. From inside, he retrieved a thermometer, stethoscope and blood pressure cuff with a rubber pump at the end. He hung the stethoscope round his neck. 'It was good timing. The note was found just as I'd finished clinic!'

'I wish I'd known you were coming, though. You nearly gave me a heart attack, showing up here like that!'

'I knew you wouldn't have called if it wasn't urgent. And I was hardly going to send a telegram.'

'This morning, when I saw you in theatre, you seemed rather cool with me. I was worried—'

'I was busy. Really, Kitty, the operating theatre is not the place for idle chit-chat.' He seemed to have put an end to any heart-to-heart she might have wished for. 'Let's tend to the patient, shall we?'

As James went about examining her sleepy mother, Kitty walked to the window and looked down at the street below. James's black Ford Anglia was parked outside the shop, now surrounded by the neighbouring children who hadn't been evacuated, together with a few nosey housewives, clutching their babies on their hips as they looked through the driver's side window and exchanged scurrilous gossip with one another – almost certainly debating if Elsie Longthorne would live or die by the end of the week. She pressed her hand to her heart where it ached the most and turned round to face the man she loved.

'Well?'

He was listening to her mother's chest through his stethoscope, wearing a sombre expression, his brow furrowed in concentration. Finally, he removed the earpieces and pressed his lips together. 'She's really rather poorly. It's good you sought medical advice without delay. A hospital would have made more sense but' – he raised an eyebrow – 'she's running a dangerously high temperature and her chest is rattling.'

'Is it a growth, do you think?' Kitty said softly, barely daring to utter the words. 'Or TB?'

He shrugged. 'I need to get her X-rayed and have her sputum and blood tested, but I'd put money on it that she's got a bad infection. Ideally, she needs some of those antibiotics we use at Park Hospital, Kitty. Except you and I both know the only patients currently allowed penicillin are military ones.'

'But the war's over!' Kitty said, balling her fist and feeling tears threaten anew. 'Surely Mam won't have to rely on sulphonamides now. Everyone knows they don't work half as well as the new antibiotics.'

James packed his bag away methodically and seemed to study a prized framed photo of Ned on her mother's night-stand – the young enlisted soldier, posing in a brand-new uniform that was too big for him. He bit his lip. 'I'll write her a prescription for sulphonamides, obviously. Though if I'm right in thinking it's an infection, it's quite advanced. I could tell you the sort of dosage she'd ideally need, if you were to get hold of some, er . . .' He didn't finish the sentence but his intention lingered in the stale air. 'Get the windows open, of course. Rest and fresh air are a must.'

Kitty smiled wryly. 'Are you suggesting what I think you are, James Williams?'

James's dark eyes darted to the doorway as if to check that they weren't being eavesdropped upon. 'Get your mother in for tests to rule out TB and a tumour. But first, let's treat this as an infection. She's got a raging fever. We can't risk blood poisoning.' He winked.

Was this what medical care for ordinary people had come to? Was Kitty *really* going to have to steal penicillin from the hospital and treat her mother herself for the want of a specialist's fee? She swallowed hard.

'Whatever it takes.'

Chapter 7

'How long have I been asleep?' her mother asked, later that afternoon. She wiped her mouth with a trembling pale hand, looking disoriented.

Kitty set her novel on her lap and smiled. 'A good three hours.' She slipped the book into her handbag and approached the bed, stroking her mother's hair from her forehead. 'You must need it, Mam.'

Her mother started to wheeze, and the wheezing quickly deteriorated into a rattling cough. She tried to sit up.

'Hang on, Mam.' Kitty helped her to get comfortable and handed her some tablets with a glass of water. 'Have a sip of water first, to stop the cough. Then take these tablets. Dr Williams came out to see you while you were asleep. He left you a prescription. I nipped out to the chemist.'

Her mother sipped the water but pushed the tablets away, shaking her head. 'I don't need none of that. I'll be right.'

'Oh, but you won't. And you're not a doctor.'

'You'll be out of pocket. That's the last thing I want on my conscience.'

'Dr Williams examined you as a favour to me. Take the pills! I insist.'

Eventually, Kitty persuaded her mother to take the medicine. Her thoughts then turned to quite how much trouble she'd be in if she didn't get back to the nurses' home soon. 'Listen, I'm going to have to skedaddle or I'll end up

50

getting the push.' She chuckled, trying to sound as bright and breezy as possible though her stomach felt like it was being squeezed tight by the devil. 'Matron thinks *I'm* the one who's ill! I only came out to tell you about Dad getting out of nick. He's the last of my worries right now, though.'

'Don't you fret over me or that rotter, Kitty, love,' her mother said, taking Kitty's hand and stroking rough, well-scrubbed skin. 'You get yourself back to Davyhulme. That's where you belong. Mixing with the likes of Dr Williams and that Violet. Lay with dogs, you get fleas. Mix with Chanel Number 5, and you'll come up smelling of it. Right?'

'I'll be back in the morning before my shift starts, I promise. I'll make you a bite to eat, if you're up to it.'

With a heavy heart, Kitty left her mother alone in the dank bedsit, praying that the medicine would work its magic overnight.

Having successfully slipped back into the nurses' home, evading detection by the matron for ditching the end of her shift, Kitty woke the following morning at 4.30 a.m. and hastened back to Hulme. She hitched a ride with the milkman, enjoying the post-war dawn sun on her face as the pony and cart trotted along the main road into Trafford. He dropped her within a mile of Mrs Ainsworth's corner shop.

'There you go, love,' the milkman said. 'I hope your Mam's back on her feet sharpish.'

'Ta! And thanks for the lift.'

He reached behind him and took a pint of milk from a crate. 'Here you go.'

'But I've not got any coupons for milk.'

'My treat,' he said, smiling and winking. 'The boss won't lose any sleep over one "broken" bottle.' He tapped on his lower leg, which sounded solid – clearly prosthetic. 'If it weren't for you angels, I might never have survived the war!'

Kitty walked the rest of the way, carrying a pint of fresh milk. She passed a bakery, just opening, and bought a National Loaf. Finally, she arrived at Mrs Ainsworth's corner shop just as she was opening up to take delivery of the day's newspapers.

'You're up with the lark,' she said, pulling her tweed overcoat closed over her nightie.

Did she ever take off that gruesome hair net, Kitty wondered? 'I've come to check on Mam. How did she do overnight?'

Mrs Ainsworth shrugged and shuffled in her carpet slippers back inside. 'I looked in on her when I went to bed, but I've not been up since. She's not my family. They'll be queueing round the block before long, all waving ration books in my face and asking for their weekly cuts of bacon and cheese; fighting over the powdered egg. I've just had a delivery of tinned peaches too. Mayhem. That's what it'll be. I can't be playing nursemaid for the lodger when I've got a business to run.'

Kitty had to bite her tongue to stop a heated response from pushing its way through her lips like a jet of scalding steam. 'Just as well you unlock early, isn't it?' She pushed past Mrs Ainsworth to the living quarters beyond the counter and climbed the stairs.

'Mam?' she whispered, knocking gently on her mother's door.

There was no response. Kitty gingerly turned the knob and pushed the door open to find her mother splayed diagonally across the bed with the covers on the floor. The fabric of her nightie was stained dark around the armpits and collar. A sheen of sweat covered her pale, pale face and there was blood on her pillow and mouth.

'Oh, blimey. This is no flipping good!' Kitty said, lifting her mother back onto the bed properly.

Her mother's eyes flickered open. She smiled weakly. 'Kitty. I was dreaming of you.'

Kitty felt her brow. 'You're still burning up, Mam. That medicine's not working.' She spoke quickly – the fear that her mother might die squeezed her throat tight until her voice became almost a squeak. 'We need to get you into hospital.'

Her mother shook her head vehemently. 'Over my dead body. My old dad went into the public hospital with his stomach. It was like a charnel house in there. We ended up wheeling him on a handcart to the workhouse to die. Some good that did him. I know you're a nurse and that, and I'm so proud of you, but –' She gripped the bedclothes so tightly that her knuckles stood proud like pearls. 'I'm not you. Don't make me go!' Her eyes were wide with fear.

Kitty took her mother's hot, clammy hand gently and stroked it until she relaxed her grip of the counterpane. 'I'm going to get hold of some of that new penicillin, Mam. Don't worry.'

Though her mother was dangerously ill, however, she seemed to stare through Kitty's eyes into her soul. 'That stuff's for the Yank soldiers, I heard you saying. What are you planning to do? Rob the hospital?' Her words were punctuated by that ominous grinding, rattling cough. 'And then you get caught and lose your job and everything you've fought for? Not on your Nelly, young lady! Not on my account.'

'Come on, Mam! Meet me halfway! You won't go into hospital. You don't want medicine I could lay my hands on easily. Listen, if you don't get proper treatment, you're going to die!'

'Better I die than you lose your future. I'm not having another Longthorne doing time. Promise me you won't steal from the hospital. Promise!'

Kitty bit her lip to stifle a wail of despair and frustration.

'I promise.'

Chapter 8

'I'm looking for Bert Longthorne,' Kitty told the dishevelled-looking man who leaned against the wall of the pub, trying and failing to coordinate his hands well enough to light a cigarette. 'Have you seen him? Is he inside? In his forties. Medium build. Grey hair and thick black eyebrows. Big mole on his nose. You can't miss him.'

'Eh? Bert who? Never mind that. How about a kiss?'

Judging by the fumes on his breath, it was clear she was wasting her time with the drunk, and time was a precious commodity she had little of, with Matron still believing her to be tucked up in bed with debilitating stomach cramps.

She pushed her way through the glazed doors into the ramshackle Victorian pub. The yellowed lounge bar was a fug of thick cigarette and pipe smoke that stung the back of her throat. The clientele was almost exclusively elderly men, stooped over their ale, though their rheumy eyes were suddenly bright, sharp and fixed directly on her. With every step she took from the door to the bar, the sticky floor seemed reluctant to let her shoes go. A surly barman was standing by the beer pumps, wiping glasses out with a grimy rag. He watched her approaching with undisguised suspicion on his pasty face.

'Sorry to bother you. Have you seen a feller called Bert Longthorne?' Kitty asked, trying to shake off the feeling that the old men were closing in on her. 'Medium build. Grey hair. Bushy black eyebrows. Mole—'

'You're a long way from home, love,' the barman said, leering her way. He licked his lips. 'Can I do you a sherry?'

'No thanks.' Kitty turned round to the other men. 'Anyone? Have you seen Bert Longthorne?'

She might as well have been talking to a pub full of ghosts. Not a single drinker acknowledged her presence. They just stared at her in glum silence until one middle-aged man staggered towards her, slurring his words as he spoke.

'How much, love?' He winked.

Realising that he'd mistaken her for a prostitute, Kitty hastily made for the exit, only slowing her pace when she was a good couple of hundred yards down the street. Her heartbeat raced; her breath was ragged.

'Pull yourself together, Kitty Longthorne,' she whispered beneath her breath.

She had two hours before her new late shift began. No matter how uncomfortable an experience this would prove to be, she had to find her errant father.

Walking through the rubble of Hulme, Kitty realised the scale of the desolation that years of bombing had brought on the area. Vast tracts of wasteland now lay where street upon street of Victorian slum terraces had once stood like brick-built platoons, standing to attention in poker-straight lines. Manchester was in tatters and, as she entered the next grimy pub that had been left standing when all else around it had been flattened by the Blitz, she realised its surviving citizens were too. Those who had been left behind were like the weak, yellowed weeds that clung to life in the cracks of the rubble. Surely, peacetime would bring hope and change for the better to the ordinary folk. Surely, things would get better for her family!

'Have you seen Bert Longthorne?' she asked a familiar-looking man in the pub that had once been her father's regular watering hole. He held a pint of soapy-looking beer with his only hand. The left sleeve of his old jacket had been pinned around the back. A war veteran, perhaps, or else a civilian casualty of the Luftwaffe's wrath.

The man shook his head. 'I haven't seen Bert since he got his collar felt for the Dunlop job. I don't think he'd be too welcome in here, anyhow. He's nowt but a malingerer and a coward. Who's asking?'

Kitty left without explaining herself, feeling the heat of embarrassment in her cheeks.

She searched the pubs of Trafford until her feet were blistered, finally reaching the outskirts of the city centre. Just as she was about to give up her quest, she found her father in The Peveril of the Peak – a tiny shining emerald of a place that had miraculously been left intact in its art nouveau green-tiled glory. He was leaning against the old mahogany bar, holding court with his fellow drinkers, who were all laughing raucously at some joke he'd just told.

'At last,' Kitty said, tugging him by the sleeve towards the door amid mocking jeers and wolf whistles from the other men. 'Come on. I want a word with you.'

'I thought you didn't want owt more to do with me,' he said, dragging hard on his cigarette. 'You've changed your tune.'

'I've got a way you can make amends.'

'Oh aye?' Her father looked at her through narrowed eyes. A smile played around his chapped lips.

She marched him up the street. Looking all around for possible eavesdroppers, she brought them to a halt in the doorway of an old empty Victorian building that had been left standing. 'Can you get something for me on the black market?'

Those sharp brown eyes were appraising her. 'I'm a reformed character,' he said, lighting a new cigarette off the glowing embers of his spent one. 'I don't do that sort of thing anymore.'

'Pull the other one. It's got bells on.' Kitty swallowed hard, knowing what she was about to ask of him was wrong. If her father were ever to lead the life of a law-abiding man, handling stolen goods was the last thing he should contemplate. But her mother's needs were acute and her father was something of a lost cause or else he'd have been searching for work, rather than propping up the bar in the Peveril. 'I need penicillin.'

'Eh? You work in a hospital! Isn't that coals to Newcastle? Wait a minute. Are you ill?' He took her arm and pulled her close, examining her face with the keen eyes of a parent.

'It's for Mam. Please.' Kitty swallowed the lump in her throat.

'Your mam's ill?'

She nodded.

'How ill?'

'If she doesn't get penicillin, she could die.'

'But you work in a building full of quacks and medicine.'

'There's only soldiers can get it on prescription at the moment. The Government still hasn't changed the rules.' She pulled herself free of his grip.

'Nick it, then. Nobody'll notice if you slip some in your apron.'

Kitty shook her head. 'Mam made me promise not to. She doesn't want me losing my job. She doesn't want me turning out like . . .' She let the implication hang in the air and looked down at her own well-scrubbed hands, chewing the inside of her cheek; angry that she should resort to this skulduggery. 'That's why I've come to you. I don't want you thieving it. If you get caught, you'll go straight back to prison. But I thought you, of all people, could find out where to get some . . . off the back of a lorry, like.'

Her father straightened up, suddenly looking a good four or five inches taller, shedding his air of desperation. 'Turns out I can provide for my family, after all.' He reached out to put his arm around her.

'Don't push your luck,' she said, taking a step back.

He held his hands up in a gesture of surrender. 'One step at a time, right? I understand. When do you need it by?'

'Yesterday.'

Her father's brow furrowed, then. 'I'm not a miracle worker, Kitty, love. I've only been out of the clink for three days. It's going to take a while to find the people in the know.'

She lowered her voice and spoke with a conspiratorial air, hating the thrill of the subterfuge. 'There's a truck delivers medical supplies to the hospital tomorrow morning.' She told her father the address of the supplier's depot, making him repeat it until he'd committed it to memory. 'The truck always arrives at Park Hospital first thing. Maybe the driver knows of some penicillin going begging . . . for a price.'

'And where do I get money for bribery?'

'I don't care how you do it, Dad, but get that penicillin to me *without delay*. We're relying on you. For once in your life, *don't* let us down.'

'She can't really be that poorly!'

Sharp words of resentment clawed their way up Kitty's throat. 'Well, she is. Right? If Mam hadn't had to work so flaming hard while you were in prison, maybe she wouldn't have got so run down. If she doesn't make it, or this turns out to be TB, the blame lies with you.' She poked him hard in the chest, torn between overwhelming gratitude that someone was there to help her and bitterness on her mother's behalf. 'I'm on nights this week. I get off shift at six. Meet me under the hospital clock tower. Wear a hat in case matron sees you and recognises you. I'll walk right past and pretend I don't know you. Follow me, but don't get too close. I'll lead you to a quiet spot where we won't be seen. You can give me the medicine then.'

With her father's assurances and some hope in her heart, Kitty made her way back to the fresh air and leafy surrounds of Park Hospital. Knowing she could only rely on women's problems as an excuse to stay away from the ward for a day or two at most, she realised it was time to report for her late shift. As she did so, she couldn't help but wonder if she'd be able to save her mother's life without ruining her own.

Having donned her uniform, Kitty marched up to the brick-and-sandstone hospital, elegant with its 1920s clean lines. She glanced up at the clock on the tower to check that she was on time. There were just over twelve hours until she was to meet her father in the early morning shadows beneath it. Would his criminal mission succeed?

Pulling her cape around her, Kitty swallowed hard, gritted her teeth and marched on to the hospital entrance, not noticing the shadowy figure at the window, watching her every move.

Chapter 9

'Are you all right?' Violet asked. She slammed the door of her locker shut almost too quickly, blushing, as though she had some secret memento hidden inside that she didn't want Kitty to see. 'You've seemed distracted the past few days.'

'I'm fine.' Kitty removed her cape and hung it on her hook. She checked that her nurse's watch was adequately wound, closed her own locker and said a silent prayer that her mother was coping in that horrible bedsit. How she wished that Mrs Ainsworth had a telephone in the shop.

'You look peaky too,' Violet said. 'Are you sleeping?'

'No. Yes. Look, we've got a long shift ahead of us and we'd better hurry before Matron has our guts for garters.'

Violet smoothed her red hair beneath her nurse's cap with a well-manicured fingernail. She treated Kitty to a wide, pearly toothed smile. 'I wondered if your late-night visitor had kept you awake.' She winked. 'That was all rather dramatic, wasn't it? Me sneaking in after curfew and you, looking like you'd lost a pound and found a penny! What a pair we are.' Her blue eyes widened. Even though she was about to start a shift, it was clear she'd darkened her eyelashes and eyebrows carefully with soot.

'I don't want to talk about it, Vi. In fact, there's nothing to talk about. That man was just a down-and-out. It had nothing to do with me.' Kitty blushed and cleared her throat, hoping to draw a line under the awkward conversation. How much had Violet heard of the exchange between Kitty, her father and Matron? It didn't matter. It was none of Violet's business. A rich girl like her wouldn't understand Kitty's predicament in any case. 'I wonder if there've been any new admissions,' she said, desperately trying to change the subject.

'But you said he was your father. Didn't I hear you say that? I could have sworn—'

'How did your VE day date go?' Was there anything Kitty could say to deflect Violet's curiosity?

'My new dress proved very popular.'

'And . . .?' Kitty had a sudden vision of Violet giggling at a joke James had intended solely for her ears. She batted the thought aside, remembering how he had loyally come to her mother's aid.

'I do love parties. I've missed them so. The war's been so dreary.'

They padded down the corridor towards the ward that would be the centre of their world until the sun rose on a new day. There definitely seemed to be a spring in Violet's step, but she was giving little away.

'Ah. Here we are!' Violet pushed against the doors to the ward, peering through the small glazed windows. 'Oh, gosh.' Her cheeks glowed pink. 'Dr Williams is talking to Matron.' Violet touched her nurse's cap. The glee in her eyes was undisguised for a split second, but then she seemed to remember that Kitty had had feelings for the young doctor from the first day that her training had begun. Her smile faltered. 'Are you going to say hello to him? He was a little brusque with you the other day, in theatre.'

'Oh, I'm not going out of my way,' Kitty said, walking on ahead. 'I've spoken to him since.' She didn't turn around to gauge Violet's reaction but she saw her friend's look of consternation reflected in the glass of a storeroom door that had been left open at a telling angle.

It told Kitty everything she needed to know. Violet was sweet on James too. Was it possible that he was the man she'd been secretly dating? She felt the blood drain from her cheeks. Could this explain the cool manner James had adopted recently whenever Kitty was around them both? *No matter*, Kitty thought, willing herself to find strength from within. *If James's allegiances have changed, I'm just going to have to take it on the chin.* She felt an ache in her chest, remembering the times they'd sat together on their all-too-few dates, gazing into each other's eyes; how lights had popped like fireworks on the insides of her eyelids, when they'd held hands in the darkness of the cinema. Every fibre of her being had celebrated what she'd assumed was the beginning of a true romance with the man of her dreams. How wrong she'd been! It had clearly never been more than companionship for him. *I always knew he was too good for me, and he was. Now, it's my mam who needs my full attention. What James and Violet do is none of my business.*

'Are you quite all right, Longthorne?' Matron asked as Kitty approached the desk. 'You look a little . . . bleary.'

Kitty bit her tongue hard, willing herself not to cry. 'The spring blossom is playing havoc with my sinuses, matron.' She smiled curtly at James. 'Dr Williams.'

He nodded at her, his dark eyes softening. Kitty felt that some unspoken understanding passed between them. When Violet caught up, however, the skin of his neck reddened, just above his collar and tie.

Blinking hard, James looked at his shining shoes. 'Ladies, I must continue my, er, rounds. I-I'll leave you in Matron's capable hands.'

'Bye, Dr Williams!' Violet shouted after him.

'Goodbye, Jones.' James turned back, making fleeting eye contact with Violet. The ghost of a smile pulled at the corners of his mouth. He must have felt Kitty and the matron watching him, though, because he turned away quickly, pushed through the double doors and was gone.

'Right, girls.' Matron lifted her winged spectacles onto her forehead and scanned a sheaf of notes attached to the clipboard in her hand. She sniffed hard in a business-like fashion and pursed her lips. 'So, Glen Hudson in bed seven has deteriorated since you were last on. He's got suspected septicaemia.'

Kitty registered a painful pang of woe in her chest at the news of her favourite patient's worsening condition. She peered over at the bookish young airman, shivering beneath his sheet.

'An amputation below the knee scheduled for nine o'clock this evening in bed ten,' Matron continued. 'And second-degree burns came in this morning in bed twelve. The rest are stable, though Tobias Delaware in bed three won't stop crying and wakes with night terrors, poor lamb. He's been sedated, but you might want to top him up if things get rowdy.'

'What is he in for again?' Kitty asked, trying to memorise all the information.

'Perforated bowel. Perforated by a bullet, that is.' Matron's nostrils flared. It was the only reaction she ever showed to the soldiers' suffering. 'He has shrapnel injuries to the neck and face, too, though Dr Williams has worked his magic, there, with Nurse Jones's famous hair!'

Violet beamed at the Matron but was met with a stony grimace.

'Only time will tell how it heals,' Matron said, turning to survey the ward full of suffering men.

The shift seemed to pass by so slowly that, at one point, Kitty was tempted to stand on a chair and take the large ward clock off the wall to see that it was, in fact, working. Methodically and dutifully, she worked with Violet to change bedpans, strip soiled sheets, renew foetid, spent dressings, mop floors and wipe bedframes. Before lights out, together with stern Sister Iris, they administered all the prescribed medication.

Standing by bed seven, Kitty looked down at Glen, who lay perfectly still. His skin was deathly pale beneath purple mottling. A sheen of sweat covered him and glistened in his hair. Setting down the kidney dish that contained the syringe and dose of penicillin that she was due to give him, Kitty gently raised her patient's eyelids and shone her pocket light in his eyes. His pupils dilated but she could see that he was dangerously ill. Cleansing his skin and filling the syringe with the thick medicine, Kitty felt a pang of guilt that her father was poised to steal from the wholesaler. But then, was it fair that her mother should be denied the chance to recover because of some health ministry edict that was now outdated?

Glen groaned and whimpered in his slumber as she slowly plunged the antibiotic into his arm. She sat beside him and said a silent prayer that he'd recover and make it home to his family across the Atlantic, though she knew from the mottling on his skin and his rapid, shallow breathing that death was standing over him, waiting impatiently.

Briefly, her young patient came to and reached out to her. She took his clammy hand.

'Nurse.' His lips were cracked and dry; his voice, hoarse.

'Take it easy, lovely,' she whispered, mopping his brow with a cool cloth. She moistened his lips with a wet cloth.

'It hurts, nurse.' He grimaced and gasped.

'I know, chicken. I know. I'm going to fetch you some more morphine – right this minute.' She tried to pull away, but he wouldn't let go.

'I'm dying.'

She shook her head firmly. 'You're going to be right as rain, Glen Hudson. You'll see. We'll finish that Hemmingway book together by the end of the week. Now, try to rest while I get you that morphine.'

'No!' His eyes were barely focussed, as though he was already looking at what lay beyond this world. 'Nurse.'

'What is it, chuck?'

He started to cry silently. 'You think a guy like me can meet a girl in heaven? Only, I know I'm gonna die and I ain't never kissed a girl before.' His breathing suddenly became even more laboured, his spirit seeming to slip further and further away with every second that passed.

Kitty knew there was nothing else she could do for him as a nurse. Yet, there was one last thing she could do for him as a human being. Fighting back her own tears, she looked over her shoulder, checking that nobody was watching except for the ever-wakeful, heavily bandaged burns victim in the next bed. She stroked Glen's cheek, leaned in and kissed him gently and chastely on the lips.

'Now you have, Glen Hudson. Now you have. Rest easy, lovey. Be at peace.'

The distance between Glen's ragged breaths grew, and presently, Kitty realised that after one long, rattling wheeze, he simply didn't breathe again. The shine had gone from his eyes. She gently closed his eyelids.

Kitty thought of Ned as she pulled Glen's sheet over his face and made a note of the time of his death on his records. It wasn't unusual for her to lose patients, but Glen's passing cut deeply – perhaps because he'd reminded her so much of her own twin. Poor, poor Glen.

Dabbing at her eyes, she looked up to find the lad with the terrible facial burns looking in her direction. His handover notes had said he was a recent admission and that his entire head had been bandaged by the nurses on the previous shift. Now, only one watchful eye peeped through the dressing. The intensity of his gaze made the hairs on Kitty's arm bristle. She yanked Glen's curtain shut and offered him a weak smile, pushing her own biting grief aside.

'Do you need anything?' she asked, moving round to his bed.

He shook his head in silence.

'Are you in pain?' Glancing at the clipboard at the end of his bed, she saw his name was Dwight Marshall, he was twenty-three and he'd been given morphine, prescribed by James.

Again, he shook his head in silence, and though Kitty felt a strange frisson of curiosity when she looked at him, she had no option but to move on to her other patients. Perhaps when the lad's burns had begun to heal, she could find out his story and keep him company a while in her few spare moments.

Chapter 10

'I'm absolutely shattered,' Violet said, flinging herself onto the chair behind the makeshift desk. She ran her fingers along the polished wooden desktop, balanced atop the bath in the infrequently used ward bathroom, which doubled as the Sister's office. Sister Iris had left in search of the consultant urologist.

'You're telling me!' Kitty agreed in a half-whisper. 'My back's broken.'

At four o'clock in the morning, the lights were low on the ward. The sound of snoring was punctuated only by the odd wail from a patient whose sleep was disturbed by nightmares. The smell of disinfectant pervaded the place. For now, they had done all they could to alleviate the suffering of their charges.

'The night shift's always a killer!' Violet said.

The balls of Kitty's feet were burning and her calves were almost in spasm from standing for so long. She stealthily took a visitor's chair from the side of a sleeping soldier's bed and carried it in, setting it beside the desk, kicking off her shoes and relishing the feel of the cool linoleum on the soles of her feet.

'Not long now.' Two hours until she was to meet her father beneath the clock tower. Would he have the pilfered penicillin? Had her mother made it through the night?

'Are you going to see the new Ray Milland film, when

it comes out?' Violet asked, pulling open the drawer in a small cabinet and having a good rummage through Sister Iris's things. '*The Lost Weekend*. That's the name. Jayne Wyman's going to be in it, too. I read about it in a Yankee cinema magazine I got from one of the GIs at Burtonwood.'

'Keep your voice down,' Kitty whispered. 'And yes. Probably. Why? Do you fancy a night at the flicks?'

'Oh, no. I've got a beau for that sort of thing,' Violet said, smiling enigmatically.

Kitty could tell that Violet was itching to be quizzed about her love life. But she was hardly in the mood to listen to Violet boast about courting some US air force officer, and the last thing she wanted was to hear that her friend was dating James. It was a relief when the creaking door heralded the return of a grim-faced Sister Iris, accompanied by the consultant urologist for the soldier who was dangerously ill with a kidney infection.

Forced to busy herself for the remaining two hours, Kitty breathed a sigh of relief when her shift was over. She yawned dramatically, though she'd never felt more awake, and took her leave from Violet.

'See you this evening!'

'Where are you dashing off to in such a hurry? You seem terribly agitated!'

'Bed, of course!'

'I'll walk back with you, then.'

How could she shake her overly inquisitive friend off? 'No. You're all right. I've got an errand I need to run, first.'

'At six in the morning?'

Kitty nodded. How on earth was she to meet her father by the clock tower if Violet was dogging her every step?

'Before you go, Jones, I'd like a word about your eyelashes,' Sister Iris said, much to Kitty's delight.

Without further delay, Kitty squeezed her friend's arm and raced out of the ward. Her heart beat so wildly, she was certain the tremors would knock the sleeping patients from their beds. But when she emerged into the early morning drizzle, clutching her cape around her, there was no sign of her father.

'Blast! This is typical,' she said beneath her breath, peering around to see if he was lurking in a bush.

Her mother was going to die if she didn't get the miracle drug. Of that she was certain. It was no use. She was going to have to go back inside and steal some from the stockroom, and if she got caught, she got caught. The last thing she was prepared to do was sacrifice her own mother for the sake of a job and a promise.

Turning on her heel, she marched back towards the hospital's entrance.

'Hang about, Kitty!' a man's voice said.

Kitty turned to a thick, tall bush and realised her father was hiding behind it. She could barely speak with excitement and dread. 'Well?' She checked the windows above for eavesdroppers and spies.

He nodded. 'Not here,' he said.

'You got it?!' Kitty said, shivering in the shadow of the nurses' home with adrenalin.

'Aye. Of course! I'm Bert Longthorne. I can get anything your heart desires, cocker!' He withdrew a rattling draw-string bag that contained the bottles of penicillin.

Kitty reached out to snatch them from him, calculating that she'd probably be able to hitch a ride into Hulme from someone driving from Urmston to one of the factories in Trafford – she didn't stand a chance of catching a bus at such an early hour.

Her father, however, had other ideas. He swung the bag out of reach, holding it aloft like a playground bully, teasing a little girl. 'Not so fast. You only get this on one condition.'

Narrowing her eyes, Kitty calculated all the different demands her father might unreasonably make on her and her mother in return for the medicine. None of them would be palatable. 'Which is?'

He opened his mouth to answer but Violet's voice sliced through the tension. She was approaching fast with another nurse, reminiscing loudly about the time Glenn Miller had come to the hospital to entertain the US air force patients. They rounded the corner.

'Kitty!' Violet said, clasping her chest. 'My word. You gave me a fright. What are you doing, just standing around?'

Blinking fast and feeling like the earth was about to swallow her whole, Kitty reached for an explanation but found none. 'I, er . . .'

'Well, are you coming inside, then?' Violet looked at her quizzically and turned to her companion, Alice Struthers, who worked nights on the TB ward. She raised an eyebrow and rolled her eyes.

In her peripheral vision, Kitty could see no sign of her father. Where had he gone? *Think of an excuse, for heaven's sake! Fob them off!* the voice in her head yelled. She surreptitiously put her hand beneath her cape and pulled her nurse's watch off her uniform.

'I can't. I've lost . . . I'm looking for my, er –' she slid the watch down into her pocket – 'watch. I must have dropped it en route from the hospital.' Kitty waved her hand dismissively and smiled. 'Get yourselves to bed, girls. I'll be along in a tick.'

She offered up a silent prayer that Violet and Alice wouldn't insist on helping her to search for the watch.

'See you, then!' Violet said, dragging Alice along with her. 'Hope you find it!'

Waiting until her two colleagues had gone inside, Kitty leaned over and grabbed her knees, barely able to breathe with fear that she'd almost been caught.

'That was close,' her father said, suddenly standing by her side.

'Where did you go?' she asked. 'How did you—'

He tapped the side of his nose conspiratorially. 'Just call me Houdini.'

Remembering the urgent task in hand, Kitty reached for the bag of penicillin yet again, but for the second time, her father held it out of reach.

'What do you want, Dad?' she asked, not hiding the irritation and frustration from her voice.

'I'm coming with you. I want to speak to your mam.'

'No! Absolutely not. Stay away from her. She doesn't want anything to do with you.'

'Like it or not, Kitty, love, I'm her husband. You want this medicine? Then I'm coming with you.'

Chapter 11

Two weeks passed, and Kitty was relieved to see her mother responding to the penicillin. As the Longthorne women woke from one nightmare, however, a new one immediately took its place. Her father was back, and it took him only days to wedge his feet firmly back under Kitty's mother's table.

'I saved your life,' he'd said, as her mother had lain in bed, laid low and vulnerable with infection. 'But that's the least I can do for the woman I love.'

At first, he'd agreed to visit only under Kitty's supervision. He'd brought an impressive bouquet of purple and white flowers, which looked suspiciously like they'd been stolen from a fresh grave in Southern Cemetery. As Kitty's mother had begun to respond to the antibiotics, she'd scoffed at his attempts to make amends. But the honeyed overtures had dripped from his tongue, as though he'd spent his years in prison writing love poetry. Every day, he'd shown up wearing fresh clothes; his hair newly shorn and gleaming with Brylcreem. The stink of stale beer had been cleverly masked with a gargle of strong-smelling TCP and cologne – not clever enough to escape Kitty's notice, though. It was clear that by the start of the second week, Kitty's mother's resolve had started to weaken.

'Oh, Bert! I've missed you. How can I ever repay you?' she'd said, taking his hand into hers.

Kitty had been able to see how her father had begun to manipulate her mother. She'd had to intervene.

'I don't think you should visit Mam anymore,' she'd said, as she'd frog-marched her father from Mrs Ainsworth's shop. 'We appreciate what you've done, but she's on the mend now. She doesn't need you in her life.'

Her father had rounded on her, then, wearing a decidedly bristly expression on his clean-shaven face. Grabbing Kitty by her elbow, he'd pulled her close – too close for comfort, with his fingers digging into her flesh. 'Listen, young lady! Last time I looked, I was your damned father.' His few tobacco-stained teeth were set in a grimace – rusting prison bars at the gateway to a hurtful hellhole of a mouth. 'Since when did you become the head of this family? You want taking down a peg or two, you do, Miss Hoity Toity. You always did think you were too good to be a Longthorne. Well, you're nowt a pound! You're just a dried-up spinster with thick ankles and ugly shoes. Know your place, Nurse Kitty, else you might find yourself joining those patients of yours in hospital!'

He'd balled his fist, his knuckles showing the pink scars of prison fights and her father's true colours. Kitty had gasped as though he had actually knocked the wind from her. She'd shaken him off and had taken several steps away from him, unable to find a response to such venom. Her father had succeeded in saving her mother's skin, only then to condemn her to a renewed life sentence of bullying and servitude. And without ever intending it, only wishing to save her mother from the grave, Kitty had colluded.

Two weeks was all it took her mother to agree to install Kitty's father in her digs above Mrs Ainsworth's shop.

'Mrs Ainsworth's going to throw you out, Mam,' Kitty said, taking her mother's temperature and blood pressure on the day before she was due back at the Ford factory. 'There's not a chance she'll put up with Dad rolling in drunk and clattering up those stairs at kicking-out time.'

'Your dad's turned over a new leaf. He promised.'

'Twenty odd years of him hammering on the door at two in the morning because he's had a skinful and locked himself out. And you think a couple of years inside will have changed him? Come on, Mam!'

'He means well. He's not causing any harm,' her mother said, rubbing her arm as Kitty removed the blood pressure cuff. She smiled weakly as though she'd already surrendered to the past.

'Oh, but he is! Can't you see it? Mrs Ainsworth has already got a face like a wet weekend every time she claps eyes on you. All because Dad keeps turning up. Believe me, Mam, taking him back is a big mistake. You're going to end up with no roof over your head, working like a navvy to keep him in beer money. How long until he's thieving again? Can you honestly see him doing an honest day's work for an honest day's pay?'

'No man'll want for a job when they all come back from the war. Mrs Ainsworth said they're going to hold a general election in the summer. Imagine if Labour get in!'

Kitty sighed long and hard. 'Labour won't get in, Mam. Churchill's bound to win and he's a Tory. Honestly, if you listened to the doctors at the hospital when they're sitting around, smoking cigars in the staffroom – the people with power in this country don't want change. The haves aren't ready to give what they've got to the have-nots.'

Her mother's lips thinned to pale slivers of pink. 'Don't

be such a Doubting Thomas, our Kitty. Clement Attlee's going to win, and we'll get everything what they put in that Beveridge Report. You'll see!'

Kitty laughed mirthlessly. 'Since when were you a political pundit?'

Her mother picked up the newspaper that Mrs Ainsworth had passed on after reading, waving it at Kitty. 'Me and the girls at work – we read the paper, you know. We listen to Pathé News. And we talk in our dinner hour. We're not behind the door with worldly matters and just because we're getting on, doesn't mean we've got nowt going on upstairs.' She jabbed at her forehead. 'And only you young'uns know what you're on about. It might be a man's war, but it's us lot what have been running the show at home.'

'Yes! Exactly. And you're prepared to let Dad back into your life so he can run you ragged and use you like a dishcloth?'

'Mind your tongue! I'm not a child and I'm not an invalid anymore.'

Kitty had had enough. The sweet relief of her mother's recovery had been embittered by her father, and she couldn't bear to hear her mother defend the disappointing bully for a moment longer.

Checking her watch, she realised that it was time to head back to the hospital for the night shift. She kissed her mother on the cheek, wishing the conversation had gone better. 'Best of luck for tomorrow, Mam. If you feel funny, take a rest. Don't push yourself. I'll be round on my day off, but if you need me in the meantime, get the receptionist at the factory to telephone the hospital and get word to me or send a telegram.'

'I've not got the money to be sending telegrams, willy-nilly.'

'And Mam –' Kitty rubbed her intractable mother's arm. 'Remember I love you and I'm here for you.'

'You can pack it in with those melodramatic overtures, our Kitty. The dark days are behind us Longthornes. Your dad's back, our Ned will come home and the family will be back together. You'll see.'

Kitty's shift began in the usual way with a mad dash to the ward, where, through the glazed doors, she could see Violet, already standing to attention by the sister's desk. Immaculately groomed as ever, as though she were stepping out to a dance, rather than beginning a gruelling twelve hours' stint spent on her feet, Violet was nodding enthusiastically at something Sister Iris had just said to the dayshift nurses. Iris now seemed to be saying something critical to Lily Schwartz, judging by the sour expression on her face. Matron was standing nearby, engaged in conversation with James, who looked as dashing as ever in his white coat.

Bursting in, Kitty smoothed down her apron. 'Sorry I'm late. I had to go all the way to Hulme to check on my mam.'

'Your personal life is of no interest to me, Longthorne,' Sister Iris said, scowling at her and folding her arms tightly across her chest. 'Your punctuality *is*, however.'

'But my mam's just recovering from a nasty—'

'I don't care if your mother's recovering from rigor mortis or a spell in Hitler's bunker. You're missing handover, and the lives of these men' – she gestured at the ward of occupied beds – 'depend on you knowing where their treatment's up to and what their individual needs are. *Don't* be late again.'

Swallowing hard, Kitty took comfort in the sympathetic smiles of both Violet and Lily.

'Don't let her upset you,' Violet whispered, once Sister Iris was out of earshot, taking instruction from Matron. 'She's a vile old bag. You should have heard what she was saying to poor Lily before you arrived!'

'She called me a snivelling little kraut!' Lily spoke behind her hand. There was a chuckle in her voice but sadness in her eyes. 'She said I was lucky I wasn't gassed or shot with the rest of "my type". Doubly insulting!'

'Iris is nothing but a big ignorant bully,' Kitty said, straightening up and trying to be strong for her colleague. 'You go home and put your feet up, Lily. Leave Sister Iris to me and Violet.'

As James was about to leave the ward, he pulled Kitty aside by the store cupboard. 'Is your mother quite recovered?' he asked, studying her face with such intensity that she was forced to look away.

'Yes. Thanks. I can get back to normality now and enjoy my nights off.' Kitty blushed, knowing that she was being brazen, dropping such an obvious hint that he should ask her out on a date.

But either he hadn't fully appreciated her suggestion, or he simply wasn't interested in her romantically anymore. 'Good, good. I hope there'll come a time in the near future when people like her won't have to worry about the cost of treatment. She was very lucky to survive. She should be jolly thankful to have a daughter as loyal as you.' He dropped his gaze to his shoes. 'Give her my best.'

People like her. His words stung Kitty as she went about her nursing duties to the extent that she was beginning to wonder if Dr James Williams's taking her to afternoon tea and offering her his coat by the shores of windy Windermere, had been but a fantasy. The truth was, people like her had nothing in common with people like him. The Longthornes were as common as muck, and Kitty felt sullied by her rogue of a father and the dire circumstances of a family that was barely clinging to its status of working class.

'The chap with the burns in bed three needs his bandages removing today,' Matron said in her ear, causing her to jump with surprise. 'But he's going to have a nasty shock when he sees what his bravery's earned him. You've a gentle way with you, Kitty. I've told Sister Iris I want you to do it.'

Kitty looked over to the young man who was always sitting up in his bed with his head turned towards her, whenever she arrived on the night shift. During his wakeful hours, she'd felt his eyes following her around the ward, though she'd never seen the naked fury of his burns revealed, since it was the nurses on the dayshift who had renewed his dressings. All Kitty had ever done for him was administer painkillers. She'd tried to engage him in conversation, but he'd never answered her back, as though combat had melted his power of speech as well as his skin. Now, she was tasked with unmasking the stranger that made the hairs on her arms stand up.

Collecting the necessary unguents to cover his newly exposed scarring, she made her way to the lad's bed, laid the kidney dish of medication on his nightstand, next to his dog tags, and checked his notes at the foot of the bed. Taking a seat on the edge of the bed, she reached behind his head and started to unravel the bandages.

'Today's the day, Dwight. Dr Williams is going to be doing reconstructive surgery on your face next week. And you're lucky, because Dr Williams is said to be second only to the famous Archibald McIndoe in East Grinstead. McIndoe's got his Guinea Pig Club with all those air force lads that got burned up with aviation fuel. He's doing amazing things with skin grafts, I hear. Well, our Dr Williams might not make headlines like him, but he's a very clever man and he'll do everything in his power to help you lead a normal life. Now, let's see what we're dealing with here.'

Her patient groaned as she removed the bandages. His face was a shiny, florid mess of mutilated skin. All hair had been singed away in whatever terrible fiery fate had befallen him. His left eye was gone and there was just a ruined eye socket. His nose was all but gone on the left side – a mere peg of angry-looking flesh. On the right side, however, most of the lad's face had been left untouched by fire. Kitty gasped. Her eyes widened as she tried to take in the unlikely sight. There was a glimmer of mischief in the lad's remaining eye, as though he'd been waiting for her reaction all along.

'Hang on a minute, mister!' she said, snatching up the dog tags from the nightstand. 'Dwight Marshall, born 1922, Cincinnati?' She read the tiny words, punched into the metal, trying to make sense of what she was reading and how it didn't correlate with what she'd seen. Leaning towards the smirking patient, she frowned and lowered her voice. 'Cincinnati, my arse!' At that point, relief mingled with wonder and annoyance. Tears started to well in Kitty's eyes, leaking silently onto her cheeks. 'Do you want to tell me how you made it out of a Japanese prisoner-of-war camp alive, Dwight? Or should I say, *Ned*?!'

Chapter 12

'Tell me it's you!' she said, shaking her head in disbelief; staring at her twin brother. 'Tell me I'm not imagining things!'

'Shut the curtains,' he whispered. His voice sounded muffled and other worldly, thanks to the damage such severe burns had inflicted on his lips.

Kitty drew the curtains sharply around the bed, never taking her eyes off the long-lost Ned. When they were hidden behind fabric and had at least the pretence of privacy, she sat beside him and took his injured hand carefully into hers – torn between wanting to rap his knuckles and throw her arms around him. Taking a deep breath, her throat was constricted by love, anger and relief when she spoke. 'All these weeks, I've been giving you painkillers and helping you onto the bedpan, and you didn't think to say it was you? *Missing in Action!* That's where we thought you were for the past *four years*. And then we get a telegram the other week, saying you're in a Japanese POW camp. What have you got to say for yourself, you – you terrible bugger? We thought you were a goner!'

'Shush! Keep your flaming voice down! I'm incognito and I'm in agony when the morphine wears off, in case you were wondering.'

'How did you get out of Japan, Ned? In fact, never mind that! How did you *end up* in Japan in the first place?'

Ned gingerly touched his face. 'Is it bad?' He winced.

'You were ugly before you went away. I'm not sure it's not an improvement, actually.' Despite her castigatory tone, Kitty tried to jolly Ned along. Given he'd been the twin who had got all the looks, he'd always been vain about his appearance. There was no doubt that when finally he looked in a mirror, he was going to be devastated by the change. 'You're going to need plastic surgery. But you're alive, and I've never been so thankful to see your lying, scheming face!'

He tried to laugh but his skin was stretched so taut across his skull, he could only chuckle half-heartedly. Kitty noticed how incredibly thin he was.

'You're skin and bone. Tell me, *Dwight*. Tell me everything.'

'I can't. Not here. I don't really want to talk about it.' He looked away.

'Who the hell is Dwight Marshall? Why are you wearing his dog tags? Why have you been admitted as a GI? We've only treated Yanks in here for a good while now.'

'It's a long story. And I owe Dwight Marshall my life – may he rest in peace. We were in the camp together at Changi, shipped out to Ban Pong. Ended up building the Burma-Siam railway. It's been—' His Adam's apple bobbed up and down in his throat. 'I don't want to talk about it, like I said. Not right now.'

'Oh, Ned. Our Ned! I can't believe you're alive. And back here, in Park Hospital, of all places. How did you wangle that?'

'Complete luck,' he said. 'It was a fluke.'

'I don't believe you. It's too much of a coincidence.'

'Don't believe me, then!'

Kitty could see her twin's irritation mounting. The story of how Ned had inveigled his way onto a ward in the very hospital where his sister worked would have to wait. 'How did you end up with such terrible burns?' She could feel a river of relieved tears welling within her, but she was so shocked by her discovery that it was almost as if the tears were drying before they reached her eyes.

'Does it matter? I'm here, aren't I?'

'The Government reckoned you were still in Japan a few days ago.'

'Well, they were fed wrong information by the Japs. I escaped months ago.'

'Escaped? Come on, Ned! Nobody escapes a Japanese prisoner-of-war camp!'

'Me and Dwight *did*. All right? Now, keep your voice down. I don't want anyone hearing!'

She reached out to touch his scarred skin. 'But these burns.'

He winced with pain, shying away from her and puffing air out of his mouth irritably. 'You don't give up, do you? If you must know, it was on the way home. We got torpedoed on a Red Cross supply ship in the Indian Ocean.'

'Oh, our Ned! Bless you. So, what's with the Dwight business? Where is your friend?'

'Shhh! Keep it down, for Christ's sake!' He paused, clearly listening out for anyone approaching. 'Poor sod never made it as far as England. He died on the ship.' Ned looked ruefully down at his bandaged hands. 'I tried to pull us both to safety but the smoke got him. I took his tags and hung them round my neck. Vowed if I made it off that boat, I'd send them to his family with a nice letter. Out of respect, like. Then there was this fireball, and all I remember after that is murderous pain and some Yanks plucking me out of the sea. When I came to, they thought I was Dwight. They'd seen the tags.'

'And wounded US airmen get transferred to this hospital, don't they?' Kitty offered, nodding slowly. 'So, you kept your gob shut and pretended to be your pal.'

'Aye. *Willy nilly, tell 'em nothing; let 'em buy a programme!* It was like God was watching over me, our Kitty. Anyway, the state of me – they wouldn't be able to tell any different.'

'Even at death's door, you're scheming, aren't you? You always were a cunning so and so, our Ned.'

'It got me back to you, didn't it? Don't be so quick to judge. But listen, our kid. My troubles aren't over. I'm still Dwight, right? Dwight from Cincinnati. Not Ned. Ned Longthorne left Manchester under a cloud.'

Kitty's stomach tightened. Though Ned's face was too sore and taut to show emotion at that moment, she could see apprehension in his remaining eye. 'Oh aye? I don't like the sound of this. Go on.'

Ned grimaced and gasped as he shuffled into a different position in his bed. 'Well, you remember that I signed up to fight in a hurry?'

'I remember it like it was last week. Mam was proud, but Dad thought you were signing your own death warrant.'

'Aye. Turns out, he wasn't far wrong. Before I went, I got in debt to some very nasty types.'

Kitty smiled, though the warm flush of happiness in her heart was being rapidly dampened by her long-lost twin's tale. 'Who?'

'It doesn't matter who.' Ned looked up at the ceiling. 'Show us my reflection, then. I'm ready.'

'You can wait,' Kitty said. 'I want to know who you're hocked up to. Is this the real reason you've assumed a dead

Yank's identity? Because you've come back and you've got to face the music? How much do you owe, Ned Longthorne? And who to?'

'Is everything quite all right, here, nurse?' Sister Iris said, sweeping the curtain aside to reveal their secret siblings' tête à tête. She glanced down at Ned's face and treated him to a sympathetic grimace.

'The patient wanted some privacy,' Kitty said, standing in front of her brother defensively. 'It's all in hand. I've just removed his bandages and I'm about to—'

Sister Iris snatched up the hand-held mirror that Kitty had stashed at the end of Ned's bed. She thrust it towards Ned. 'Here, young man. Let's not prolong the agony. It's not a pretty picture. You'll be glad of our Dr Williams's ministrations.'

Tempted though she was to knock the mirror out of the sister's hand to save her brother from heartbreak, Kitty held her tongue and took a step back. Ned needed to know what he was up against. She swallowed hard as she saw his ruined face turn from a half-smile to a picture of desolation.

'Oh,' he simply said, eyeing the angry welts on his skin, his devastated nose and empty eye socket.

'The main thing is that we keep you hydrated and avoid infection,' Sister Iris said. 'Dr Williams has had quite a few lads in like you. He'll probably start by—'

'Why don't I tell this brave fellow what I'll be doing for him?' A man's voice cut through Sister Iris's bluster, making Kitty start.

'Dr Williams!' she said, clasping her hand to her chest as she turned around to see James standing at the foot of Ned's bed.

She and Sister Iris moved aside to let the hospital's brightest surgeon approach his patient. Kitty felt a swell of pride and hope as she listened to James's plans for Ned.

'Well, Dwight,' he said, sitting on the edge of the bed. 'The good news is that I'm going to make you a new nose and, unless you prefer the pirate look, a new eye too.'

Ned continued to stare at his tragic reflection in the hand mirror in silence. He nodded half-heartedly as James went on.

'The bad news is that there's going to be a lot of surgeries scheduled for you. Perhaps as many as twenty or more. This is not like removing your appendix. The new cosmetic procedures take time and patience. Men like me who are becoming something of a specialist in the field are still learning on the job, I'm afraid. And there's an extra layer of complexity for you, Dwight. Given you're a US airman, you'll have to complete your treatment in America. But I'll refer you to a terrific surgeon over there.'

Looking at him askance with his good eye, Ned opened his mouth to say something but seemed to think better of it.

Kitty realised then the enormity of Ned's lie. He was being treated at Park Hospital as an American pilot, not a British soldier, and would be repatriated very soon back to Ohio as Dwight Marshall. How on earth could Ned leave Manchester and all that he knew, after having only just arrived back in the country from the Far East, to take on the identity of a dead man on yet another continent? Dwight's parents would know the man claiming to be their son was a fraud. Kitty was certain that Ned wasn't speaking because he couldn't successfully emulate an American accent. He'd never been good at acting. Yet, here he was, walking in a dead man's shoes towards an uncertain fate that could see him thrown into a US military prison.

'I'm going to take skin from your leg, and attach it to your nose, forming a tube that will connect to your shoulder,' James continued, oblivious to the unfathomable drama that was unfolding in Kitty's imagination. 'You'll have to get used to that for a while, because it lessens the chances of the graft being rejected and ensures we set up a good blood supply.' He chuckled – his dazzling white smile lighting up the dreary place. 'You might look like the Elephant Man for a while, but don't worry. It won't stop the girls loving you. The ladies are all partial to a war hero!' Then his handsome face relaxed into a more serious expression. 'I'll do my very best for you, Dwight. We're seeing great success with this kind of reconstructive surgery and –' he sniffed and blushed – 'if I say so myself, my glass eyes are the best you'll come across. I make them by hand and yours will be a perfect match with your healthy eye. People will hardly realise. After a while, when you've got used to the change in depth perception, you'll not give it a second thought. You'll even be able to drive.' Looking down at the high shine of his shoes, despite his apparent confidence, James seemed shy in the presence of his patient, or perhaps just ill at ease with the enormous weight of responsibility on his shoulders. Was all the doctor's bluster for show?

'That sounds very encouraging, doesn't it, Dwight?' Kitty said, taking the mirror from Sister Iris as a cue for her to leave. 'Now, I'm sure the doctor's busy and Sister Iris has other patients to check on. So, why don't I finish tending your wounds and make you comfortable for the night?'

She was desperate to get her foolhardy brother alone, now.

Finally, Sister Iris and James advanced to the end of the ward and another patient who was due surgery in the morning. Kitty dabbed at Ned's face. She spoke in a near-whisper that only he could hear.

'You've got to come clean,' she said, wincing inwardly herself, each time he gasped with pain at her touch. 'This is ridiculous. If you continue this charade, you'll get yourself into more hot water than being in debt to some local hoodlum.'

'I owe five thousand quid, Kitty.'

Kitty almost dropped her kidney dish. '*Five thousand?* But that's a king's ransom! That's more than you could hope to earn in a lifetime! How the hell did you rack up that kind of debt?'

He shook his head.

'Did the man you owe this money to . . . did he go off to war?'

'Didn't everyone?'

Kitty raised an eyebrow. 'No! A few managed to wriggle out of it, including Dad.'

A shadow seemed to pass over Ned's healthy eye.

'He's just got out of the nick, if you're wondering,' Kitty explained. 'He got lifted for burglary. Mam's taken him back, of course.'

'Millions dead, but it would've been too much to ask for *him* to get flattened by a doodlebug.'

'Well, we *are* talking about Dad. Anyway, maybe the man you're in debt to is dead. You'd better pray he is, because Ned Longthorne can't pretend to be Dwight from Ohio indefinitely. Are you willing to break Mam's heart? Break my heart by walking out of our lives just as you've come home? You can't afford American medical bills! They're even worse over there than they are here. At least Dr Williams will operate on you for free if we make a case for you.

Over there, you'll get found out, Ned. You mark my words. You'll end up banged up with a bunch of Yanks, who'll all want to know why the skinny Limey, with an elephant's trunk instead of a nose left their mate to die in the East. Which is it to be? An easy target in a Yank military prison or take your chances in Hulme as Ned Longthorne, war hero? And make your mind up fast, because people don't like being lied to!'

Chapter 13

Some weeks passed, and though the cast of the Longthorne family drama had been reassembled in full, Kitty had never felt more beleaguered. Thanks to her ruinous father getting his feet well and truly back under her mother's table, her mother had been ejected from the single-occupancy bedsit above Mrs Ainsworth's shop.

The ill-suited couple had been forced to move to a two-up, two-down in Chorlton-on-Medlock. It was one of only two houses left standing in the middle of a rubble-strewn bomb site, cowering in the eerie shadows cast by the skeleton remains of 'Little Ireland's' mills. The only other signs of life were the rats that scurried for cover among the piles of rubbish and the odd gaggle of barefoot children who roamed the decimated streets in search of adventure and something worth salvaging.

'You haven't even got proper sanitation, Mam!' Kitty had said, eyeing the slum dwelling with horror. Her mother had cleaned it up to the best of her ability but the place was still a death trap.

'There's running water,' her mother had said.

Kitty had glanced up at the cracks in the ceiling and walls that were big enough to fit a man's hand inside. 'It's probably not structurally sound. What if it falls down in the night and kills you? Is it worth risking your life for *him*?' She'd pointedly glared at her father, who had sat in silence on a filthy old armchair, pretending to read the paper as though he could do anything other than look at the photographs and imagine what the articles said.

'I wouldn't be alive if it weren't for your dad.'

'How long before you come down with something else and can't work – or worse?'

Her mother had gazed wistfully through the cracked glass of the window, tears welling in her eyes. 'Well, I don't need to worry about work, do I?'

'What do you mean?' Kitty had experienced that sinking feeling yet again. She'd known bad news was coming.

'I lost my job at Ford, didn't I?'

'Did they find out he's a jailbird, then?'

Her mother had shaken her head, scratching at her greying hair beneath her scarf. 'They're laying all the women off, aren't they? Now the fellers are home. They want their jobs back and us girls are all out of collar. I'm living off my coupons. And I'm on the lookout for a bit of cash in hand, if you know of anything going at the hospital or working for one of them fancy doctors. Washing, ironing, cleaning, canteen work. Anything.'

Leaving her parents' new slum dwelling, determined to find them better accommodation and to enquire after openings at the hospital for her mother, Kitty had wondered if the end of the war hadn't brought more horrors to Manchester than Hitler had himself. Now that the dust of battle had begun to settle, what she'd seen was not pretty: a woeful shortage of safe housing, even harsher rationing, surly men returned home, plagued by nightmares from the frontline and expecting their independent, capable womenfolk to revert from being the breadwinners to the roles of housewife and mother. There had been constant talk in the hospital staffroom lately about a general election being called. The consultants had sucked contemplatively on their pipes and cigars, discussing Britain's prospects in peacetime – Professor Baird-Murray the most animated and eloquent among them.

'Churchill's got it in the bag,' he'd announced to the room, adjusting his blue bow tie. 'One can't refute his wartime success. He's a leader of men, par excellence, whether at the helm of a coalition or back in his rightful place at the head of the Conservative party. It's time the Tories took back control.' He'd sunk back into his winged armchair by the wireless, regally placing an arm on each armrest, like a king on a throne. 'The last thing we need is Bolsheviks, telling us how to do our jobs and robbing us of our livelihoods, eh?'

'Hear, hear!' the other consultants had agreed, exhaling plumes of blue-brown smoke, as though they'd been old dragons, engaged in parliamentary debate as a temporary distraction from guarding their hordes.

Only James had dared to disagree, folding his arms tightly across his tweed suit. Kitty had listened as he'd spoken in quiet, deferential tones, though he never broke eye contact with the hospital's most senior specialist. 'I-I'm sorry, professor, but I think you'll be surprised, come July. The country's in shreds. It was, before the war, and it's worse now. I'm no Marxist, by any stretch of the imagination, but despite the heavy toll that war's taken on our population, the poor still number in the multi-millions. Battle scarred and hungry they may be, but they're emboldened by victory, and they're remembering that they have a voice.'

'Tosh, Dr Williams!' the professor had said, straightening up. 'The common man needs to be governed by his elders and betters. 'Twas ever thus. Churchill at the head of the

Conservatives is our only hope to rebuild the great nation he saved from defeat!'

'Well, I beg to differ, I'm afraid.'

Kitty had noticed that James had been balling his fists, though he'd shoved them deeply into his armpits. The sinews in his jaw had flinched and his right foot had twitched repeatedly as he crossed his legs.

'We're long overdue reform, gentlemen,' he'd continued, ignoring the glances that the more senior consultants and surgeons had exchanged with one another. 'The Beveridge Report only served to highlight the need to vanquish our five giants of Want, Disease, Ignorance, Squalor and Idleness.'

'The lad's a bally Liberal, Cecil!' the head of orthopaedics had said, wheezing with laughter as he'd relit his pipe.

'I'll not discuss my personal politics with you, Dr Swanley. Though I am trying to make the point that if Churchill doesn't succeed because the common man sees a Labour government as representing his interests better, don't be surprised. Beveridge's National Health Service may yet see the light of day. I, for one, can only see it bringing good.'

Kitty had watched with dismay as the room had erupted into raucous laughter at James's observations. Watching all those doctors, who had known nothing but comfort and privilege in their lives, belittling the plight of ordinary folk like the Longthornes, had been hard. She'd noticed how James had blushed with indignation. He'd risen in silence and had left the room, unaware that even the senior nursing staff had gone on to join in with the other doctors' ridicule of a National Health Service *and* of Dr James Williams – its champion within Park Hospital. She, at least, valued his heroic intentions. This quiet, studious and serious man had been surprising her with his strength of character and refreshing take on a changing world since the first day they'd met, when she'd observed him holding his own in another debate with Professor Baird-Murray. Her admiration of him was unwavering, which made his recent increasingly cool demeanour towards her all the more painful.

Yes, the few weeks that had passed after Ned's revelation had brought yet more discord into Kitty's life. Despite swapping to the day shift, and inwardly rejoicing that the man she'd recklessly fallen for was principled and caring, she'd felt her spirits slump. James had started to share more meaningful looks and secretive chat with Violet, preferring to have her assist him in theatre, while Kitty was relegated to back-breaking duty on the ward with Lily Schwartz, plagued by an overly critical Sister Iris.

All the while, Violet had primped and preened at every available opportunity, boasting about her 'eligible beau' and disappearing off whenever she wasn't on duty, usually returning under cover of darkness through the kitchenette window, well beyond curfew. Kitty had more than an inkling that James and Violet had started courting, much to her chagrin, though at no point had James ever told Kitty that his interest in her had dwindled. He'd merely killed her romantic hope with stony-faced silence.

The second predicament, however, was Ned. His treatment had begun but he was still posing as Dwight from Cincinnati. Now, Kitty yanked the curtains around his bed and faced her twin brother.

'They're starting to let civilians back on the wards, Ned,' she whispered. 'Don't you think it's time to come clean about who you are?'

Ned was sitting on the bed, dressed in a donated shirt and slacks. He'd been encouraged by Matron, at James's suggestion, to eschew his hospital-issue pyjamas in favour of normal clothes. It would be a step in the direction of rehabilitation now that his surgeries were underway. Except, the sight that greeted Kitty was anything but a picture of normality or recuperation.

Touching the tube of flesh that connected his face to his shoulder, – the beginnings of a new nose, fashioned from grafted skin and ligaments that was rather reminiscent of an elephant's trunk – Ned frowned. 'I can't. I've told you. I've left it too long now.' He beckoned her close and whispered with urgency. 'You can't keep up a lie like that and then turn around and say, "Oh, I'm sorry. I've been making a fool out of you all, these past couple of months, but don't take it the wrong way, everyone! I meant well".' The sarcasm dripped thickly from his scarred mouth, the anguish visible in his one good eye.

'I just think honesty's the best policy, Ned. The longer this nonsense goes on, the worse it will be for you. Tell them you bashed your head or something and weren't thinking straight.' Kitty checked through a gap in the curtains to see that they weren't being eavesdropped upon.

'Dr Williams will stop my treatment. I'll get slung into nick. You said it yourself. I've committed fraud. If I leave this place as Ned, I'm a dead man. Damned if I do and damned if I don't.'

'What about giving your own parents some hope? Don't you think it would make our mam's day if she knew you were alive and staying a few miles down the road, instead of rotting in some prisoner-of-war camp? They still haven't liberated the other lads stuck in Japan.'

'Exactly. People'll ask questions. Questions I'm not prepared to—'

Kitty was startled when the curtain was swept aside to reveal James, standing at the foot of Ned's bed with a clipboard and pen. 'Dr Williams! I had no idea—'

'You look like you've seen a ghost, Nurse Longthorne.' James looked pointedly over at Ned.

Was it possible that he knew of Ned's subterfuge? How long had he been standing on the other side of the curtain? Had he been listening in to their hushed conversation? Kitty's heartbeat thundered inside her chest at the thought of being caught out.

'No ghosts here, Dr Williams. Only young Dwight, grumbling about his lunch.'

'So, you've finally given up your vow of silence, Dwight? Oh, that is good news. Perhaps you can finally tell me more about how you came to sustain those injuries. Your medical history would help, too.' James raised a dark eyebrow, but there was no hint of amusement in his expression.

For mere moments that felt like hours, Kitty stood by her twin brother, wondering what he'd say. Ned merely shook his head, however.

'Saving the chat for the girls, I see,' James said, scribbling something down on the clipboard. He turned to Kitty, those sharp brown eyes seeming to strip away her layers of artifice. 'Nurse, can I have a quick word in private please?'

Smiling weakly, Kitty's hands grew clammy. Fear prickled down her spine. As she followed James to the storeroom beyond the sister's office, she knew he was about to say something dreadful. She walked in after him, and he closed the door behind her. The air in the tiny room felt too thick to sustain them. Suddenly, Kitty was alone with the man she loved for the first time in months. Not since they had been to the cinema together and had held hands in the back row had she had her favourite doctor all to herself. Yet, she knew from the stern expression on his face that he wasn't about to reveal that he did love her after all.

He clasped his hands together. 'What's going on with that patient, Kitty? I know there's something between you. Sister Iris said—'

'It's not what you think.' Kitty swallowed hard. Should she tell the truth or keep covering for Ned?

'Oh. What precisely do you suppose I think?'

'That I've struck up some romance with a poor disfigured US airman.'

'Think again.'

'That one of your patients has told me a terrible secret about his wounds.' She studied every eyelash that fringed his eyes, every pore on his nose, every crease in his lips, wishing she could blurt out everything. Her brother's pretence. Her desperation over her mother. Her jealousy of Violet. Her longing for Park Hospital's brightest young doctor, who stood before her now, bristling with annoyance.

'I know, Kitty. I know who Dwight really is. I saw the photo of him at your mother's, remember? Not all of his face has been damaged beyond recognition. I'm not stupid.'

She bit her lip and felt the blood rush to her cheeks. 'You're still treating him.'

'I'm a doctor. I don't differentiate between fraudsters and genuine war heroes.'

'I can explain!' She grabbed at his hand but he pulled away. 'Is this why you've been cold-shouldering me? You think I'm some sort of –' Kitty tried to find suitable words that might describe how the son of a barrister might see a low-born girl like her. 'Degenerate scum?'

97

'A liar is a thief, Kitty. You've dragged me into two dishonest deeds. I'm very disappointed. I thought you and I—'

Kitty felt the words march ahead in defiance of her brain's command. She simply couldn't halt them. 'I love you. I thought you felt the same way.'

'I thought I knew you.'

'You *do*! We can still—'

'Violet and I . . . We're . . . I intend to ask her to marry me.' He looked down at his brogues, blinking too hard and too often, seemingly unaware, or, at least, unconcerned that, in that stifling storeroom, he had broken Kitty's heart.

Chapter 14

'Blimey. It's so hot,' Lily Schwartz said, pausing to waft a little muggy air in front of her flushed face. 'I'm melting, even with the windows open.' She looked around furtively, presumably to check that Sister Iris didn't have her beady eye on them.

Kitty nodded. 'I know. It's unbearable. But at least we're not wearing a heavy cast on our legs or struggling through labour on the maternity ward. Imagine that!' She started to tuck her side of the sheet beneath the firm waterproof mattress of the hospital bed, folding the stiff cotton down at the corners with precision.

'All these beds to change and we've got time to gossip, have we, girls?' Sister Iris said in a booming voice. She was striding down the ward towards them with flat feet and an expression that could curdle the milk in her tea and melt the butter on her toast – if the July heat hadn't already done so. She was glaring through her horn-rimmed glasses at Lily. 'Come on, you two! Stop lollygagging. Now the GIs are going home, we've got local men waiting to fill these beds before the day shift's out. British ex-soldiers on their last legs, thanks to six years spent in the trenches, fighting the *Nazis*.' She scowled at Lily, as if the poor German-born nurse hadn't realised that every time Iris spat the word 'Nazis' into conversation, the insult was aimed at her and seemingly her alone.

Despite the heat, Iris paled visibly and smoothed the sheet with the flat of her hand until it was taut enough to bounce a coin on. 'Sorry, Sister Iris.'

'We're only saying how hot it is,' Kitty said, wanting to defend her beleaguered colleague but realising she could jeopardise her own career by being too confrontational with her superior. Matron had already cut her a good deal of slack and she was certain she no longer had an ally in James. 'Maybe it's election fever.'

'We're all suffering, Longthorne. But a professional never complains. Our patients have far more to grumble about and are looking to their nurses for a bright smile and a sunny disposition.' Iris's thin lips curled downwards. 'When you've finished those beds, matron wants you next door 'til two o'clock.'

'Over dinner?' Kitty asked, crestfallen at the thought that she wouldn't be able to cast her vote in the general election until the evening, when her shift had finished.

'Yes. They're short staffed. Too many swooning women with dehydration, I shouldn't wonder.' Sister Iris rolled her eyes. 'And it doesn't help that Dr Williams has called Jones away yet again to assist in theatre, plus Agnes Bickerstaff's father has just died.'

'But, I really wanted to—'

'No ifs. No buts. It's going to be bedlam on this ward later, but I can spare you 'til two. Missing a meal won't kill you. Now, get those beds changed and off you pop.'

Once the beds were prepared for the incoming patients, Kitty and Lily made their way over to the adjacent ward, where hell on earth awaited, ventilated only by half-opened windows.

'Am I seeing things?' Kitty asked, peering at the thermometer on the wall. The red liquid reached almost up to 100 degrees Fahrenheit. 'It's like an inferno in here.'

'Election fever,' Matron said, handing Kitty a list of tasks that needed to be done. 'Now, there's a good girl. Get cracking on these. We've got not one but two battered wives at the far end. One – Molly Pennington – has had her arm dislocated and is concussed, the other – Bridget O'Malley – has a broken nose. Keep your eyes peeled for their husbands trying to visit. I'll absolutely not allow aggressive men on my ward. Not while I have breath in my body.' Matron fanned herself with a red-and-black propaganda leaflet from the Labour party that showed the illustration of a smiling woman and the slogan, 'Labour for Homes'.

Kitty squinted to read the small print, *She can't make a home 'til she gets one.* A sorry image of her mother flickered into her mind's eye: Mam, trying to make the best of a house that wasn't fit for the rats and cockroaches she shared the ramshackle shell with. Professor Baird-Murray and the other senior consultants were so incredibly intelligent and worldly – far more so than Kitty could ever hope to be. They were men with letters after their names and the respect of the great and the good of the city. But despite their insistence that Churchill was the only man fit to get the country back on its feet, Kitty felt sure her vote belonged elsewhere, and that the opinions of the working man mattered. Would James be a Liberal or would he vote Labour? And how might that turncoat, Violet, vote?

Matron flapped the paper in Kitty's face. 'Are you paying attention?'

'Yes, matron.'

'Well there's a poor young lady in bed three who's suffered terrible injury after a backstreet abortion.' Matron whispered the dreaded word, mouthing each syllable with an air of melodrama. 'Of all the trauma I saw during the war, with those mutilated boys coming back from the front . . .' She paused while a gaggle of trainee doctors walked past with the chief radiologist, Sir Basil Ryder-Smith, resuming her confession only when the men were out of earshot. 'The sight of a girl, however dubious her morals, having been butchered on a kitchen table in some backstreet hovel – it still rattles my cage, even with all my years of experience.'

'Is she bad?' Lily asked, looking at the girl who couldn't have been more than sixteen.

'Let's just say she'll never have children now,' Matron said, closing her eyes emphatically. 'Doctor's stitched her up and prescribed a blood transfusion. She'll be lucky if she doesn't develop septicaemia, though, because I don't think surgical hygiene was on the mind of whatever fiend did the dastardly deed, and what she really needs is penicillin. But at least she's sleeping, now.'

'Pray for a miracle?' Lily said.

Matron's nostrils flared. 'Miracles can happen, Schwartz, though I prefer to rely on modern medicine for them, rather than God.' She turned to Kitty. 'Now, I want you to start with a bed bath for the gentleman in the next bed to her. Douglas MacLeod. He's been admitted with complications, following the amputation of his leg at a field hospital in Tripoli, poor soul. He's in surgery at four this afternoon, but he can't stay on my spotless ward as he is. Get him cleaned up. There's a good girl.'

Advancing to her charge, Kitty saw that the man was about the same age as she and Ned were. She thought about her twin fleetingly – how his treatment was progressing well and how James had said nothing more about his false identity, though he'd advised Ned to blame amnesia if he wanted to come clean and evade arrest for his duplicitous ruse. Ned was currently living with other American servicemen, who were under the care of James and his reconstructive surgical wizardry. Kitty felt her stomach tighten and realised it was a pang of guilt that James was *still* keeping the Longthornes' squalid family secrets. Small wonder he preferred the daughter of a bank manager to the daughter of an ex-convict.

'Deary me,' she said, setting down her towels and bowl of hot water on Douglas's nightstand. The stench of rotting flesh hit her and she realised the stump of his leg, amputated at the knee, had turned gangrenous. Swallowing down the bile that threatened to surface, Kitty smiled sympathetically and pulled back the sheet that covered the painfully swollen stitches. The entire area had begun to turn black. She was certain he'd lose what was left of his leg if he were to have a chance of survival. 'That's quite a war wound! Tripoli, I hear?'

The patient nodded, wiping his sweaty brow. His eyes weren't entirely focussed, Kitty noticed. He reached out and grabbed her hand, speaking hurriedly. 'The panzers are coming! It's too late! Just let me die, nurse.'

Kitty shook him loose as gently as possible and smiled. 'I'm afraid I can't do that. I'm here to make you better! You'll be feeling right as rain after your surgery. You'll see. And don't worry about those panzers. We make short shrift of those at Park Hospital. You're safe here!'

The man was clearly delirious with infection, though he seemed to have a moment of lucidity. He started to weep, shaking his head. 'I can't afford this. My family's going to be penniless. Just send me home, nurse. I'm already living on borrowed time.'

'Oh, don't you worry about money. We're not going to cart you off to the workhouse to die. Those days are over! Just you worry about getting better. How many children do you have?'

'Five. Another on the way. What kind of a father can I be to them when I'm trapped in a tank in the middle of the desert?'

'A healthy one! That's what.'

As she cleaned up her patient, Kitty gnawed at the inside of her cheek and not just to distract herself with pain from the stench of the man's infected leg. She'd given him false hope. Douglas was under the care of one of the older surgeons and it was entirely possible that, if he survived, he would indeed be given a bill. The gangrene in his leg was so advanced, that it was clear this man, who had fought for king and country, had been keeping away from the doctor for as long as possible, fearing that he would be taking bread out of his family's mouths if he paid for an appointment.

Coupled with the girl in the adjacent bed who was whimpering in her sleep after the backstreet abortion she'd endured, if this wasn't proof that the country needed reform in the way medical services were run, Kitty wasn't sure what was.

As soon as her chores were complete, Matron allowed Kitty to slip away to vote and to grab something to eat and drink before she rejoined the patients on the ward who were suffering from heat exhaustion.

Hastening to the polling station with excitement she could barely contain, Kitty joined the queue of hospital staff and locals who were waiting in the July heat to enter and mark their ballot papers with an X.

'I wonder who'll win,' one of the elderly women said, spluttering her words, thanks to several rotten teeth, standing like ancient tombstones amid florid gums. 'If Labour gets in, my Harold says we'll get a welfare state! Imagine that, Dorothy! I'll be able to see the dentist for free. Maybe he'll yank these and I'll get some nice dentures.'

Dorothy wasn't convinced and looked like she'd smelled something unpleasant. 'Churchill's never leaving Number Ten. A Tory Prime Minister is a foregone conclusion. My Alfred told me it's the only way to vote. How else are small businesses like our shop going to recover?'

Kitty knew that Davyhulme was a reasonably affluent area, compared to Hulme, but it was hard to tell from the women's conversation who would get the winning vote. It was the first time Kitty had been able to exercise her democratic right. She'd been too young to vote when the last election had been held, some ten years earlier. Now was her chance.

She was just about to enter the polling station when Violet and James emerged, laughing and holding hands.

'Hello, Kitty!' Violet said, her burnished amber hair glowing in the sun. 'We've not spoken in an age. Fancy bumping into you, here!' She released James's hand as though it were a burning coal.

'Couldn't miss my chance to make a difference,' Kitty said, wishing the ground would swallow her whole so she didn't have to see her supposed best friend and the love of her life together. She turned to James. 'Dr. Williams.' She willed the sudden wave of sadness to stay locked inside her aching chest. 'I know you're keen for reform, as am I. Best of luck!'

'Thank you, Kitty,' James said, casting a surreptitious glance her way and then looking off in the direction that the hospital lay. He stuffed his hands into the pockets of his trousers.

Violet did no such thing, however. She ran her hand through her hair, pouting playfully. 'My James is *such* a do-gooder!' Her finger glinted as she stuffed her hand through the crook of his arm, pulling him to her in her own personal Anschluss. 'Darling, if your father knew what your politics were, I'm sure the curls in his barrister's wig would droop. What would your mother's bridge friends say? What would *my* mother say?'

James cleared his throat and flashed her an uncomfortable smile. 'Oh, I don't know, Violet. Your mother rubs shoulders with theatrical folk and artists. They're famously progressive types, aren't they? They understand the plight of the common man.'

'Common like the Longthornes? The picture houses and dance halls are stuffed with the likes of your family, aren't they, Kitty? Writhing to jazz and getting hot under the collar over Errol Flynn and Bette Davis. I bet your, mam wouldn't know Puccini if *Che Gelida Manina* was sung in her front parlour.' She trilled with laughter.

'Violet! Is that really necessary?' James flashed Kitty an apologetic glance and ushered the ever-preening Violet away.

Willing herself to ignore the jibe, Kitty wondered why Violet's hand had glimmered so – then she realised. She'd been wearing a diamond ring! In fact, she'd clearly been desperate for Kitty to see that she and James were engaged to be married.

'Come on, love! Move inside!' the man behind her in the polling queue said.

'Sorry,' Kitty said, wiping tears away before anyone started to question why the plain-looking nurse with the thick ankles and sensible shoes was crying.

Taking her ballot paper to the booth, Kitty read the list of candidates. She already knew how she was going to vote, however. The nation needed more than empty promises. She marked an X in her chosen square and posted her paper into the ballot box. Hopeful for the country, though on a personal level her optimism had deserted her entirely.

Later that evening, as her arduous shift ended and she and Lily parted company, Kitty met Ned in the lounge of The Garrick's Head pub, at his suggestion. It was an impressive part-timbered old place that looked at odds with the utilitarian brick buildings in the vicinity – like Park Hospital – that had been built in the 1920s and 1930s. At dinner time on Election Day, the lounge was empty but for two or three old men and a large golden retriever. The air hung heavy with smoke and the walls were yellowed from decades of nicotine nights and draught bitter days. She spotted her brother seated in a corner on his own.

'You're brave to go out,' she said, eyeing her brother's peculiar features sympathetically.

He was wearing an eye patch and studied her with his good eye. Half of his face was still nightmarish, in spite of the recognisable beginnings of a new nose. Though still slender for a man in his twenties, he had at least lost the alarmingly skeletal appearance that he'd had on his arrival at the hospital. 'What option do I have? If I stay with the other sideshow freaks, I can't speak. They think I'm mute from shock.'

'Can't you put it on? The accent, I mean.' Kitty observed the other drinkers to check that they weren't eavesdropping. She lowered her voice. 'Surely, if you spent all that time in the prisoner-of-war camp with the real Dwight—'

'Oh, come on, Kitty! I was never good at acting.' Ned gingerly poured some beer into his damaged mouth, dribbling half of it down his shirt. He wiped his lips on his sleeve. 'One word and the game would be up! Yank military prison. They'd throw away the key, mark my words!'

Kitty snorted with derision. 'Never good at acting? And yet here you are, walking in a dead man's ill-fitting shoes because you got into hot water with some real bad'uns – which we never knew a thing about. Wide-eyed and innocent Ned, who can't act for toffee? No! Butter wouldn't melt in our Ned's mouth.' She couldn't stop the sarcasm from souring her words. 'Don't make me laugh. Your whole adult life's been a lie!'

Ned frowned, looking suddenly small and vulnerable. 'Have you come here to rub salt into my wounds, Kitty? Don't be so quick to judge. You don't know what I went through to get back to Blighty, but you do know *why* I ended up running away to the Far East in the first place. How's a lad to keep on the straight and narrow when his only role model is a thief and, now, a jailbird? Tell me!'

'I managed to avoid a life of crime,' Kitty said. 'Funny that! Do you see me on the game or living over the brush with some common criminal? Or did me and Mam manage to dust ourselves off, roll up our sleeves and graft our way out of the mire? Eh? Didn't Mam always warn you if you lie with dogs, you get fleas? She might as well have been talking to the flaming wall. I was listening, Ned. What's your excuse?'

Ned lit a cigarette and dragged the smoke deep into his lungs. He exhaled through his mouth, coughing and spluttering.

'You shouldn't be smoking,' Kitty said, grabbing the cigarette from him and stubbing it out on a well-used tin ashtray. 'How can you do that with no nose? And between surgeries too! It's dirty.'

'I didn't come here for a lecture. What do you want?'

'I want you to tell the truth. I want you to stop pretending. I want my Ned back.'

'I can't.'

'The man you owe money to. I got Dad to ask around. He's dead. Turns out, he was carted off to fight in North Africa just after you left. Killed in action. You're safe.' Kitty grabbed a bunch of the fabric of her skirt and squeezed hard, willing Ned to listen to her logic.

Ned shook his head. 'I don't believe you, and anyway, first, the man I owe money to – no way will my debt have died with him. He had pals, and they'll still see me as owing. Secondly, I'm getting my treatment for free as a Yank. That Dr Williams of yours has persuaded Dwight's commanding officer to let me stay here as a guinea pig for this plastic surgery business. If I go back to being Ned, even if I don't end up in the clink, where am I going to live? With Mam and Dad in the middle of a bomb site? Where am I going to find the money to pay for my treatment?'

'Right! That's it! I've had enough!' Kitty was hot, tired and broken-hearted. She slammed down her glass of lemonade, unable to tolerate Ned's stubbornness any longer. 'If Labour gets in, will you give up this ludicrous charade? Come on, our Ned! Would you see Mam mourn you unnecessarily if you can get treated for free by the National Health Service – if you get given a nice new place to live on Civvy Street *in peace*?'

'Labour'll never get in,' Ned said. 'You're dreaming.'

Chapter 15

'Today's the day, our Kitty!' Kitty's mother said, as they queued for food together outside Mrs Ainsworth's shop. 'By this afternoon, we'll know who's won the election. You mark my words, the twenty-sixth of July 1945 will go down in history as the day people like us finally got a say in how our lives are run.'

Kitty linked arms with her mother and advanced a couple of places towards the door, as other women shuffled inside. Her stomach rumbled loudly. 'I hope you're right, Mam. There's a lot riding on a Labour win. We should be so lucky!' She chuckled mirthlessly and looked up into the overcast Mancunian sky. It was still warm, but the sun was hiding behind otherwise bruising skies. Kitty felt like anything could happen that day. The sun might come out, or storms could just as easily lie ahead. 'I swear, if they tighten up rationing any more, we're all going to starve to death. I'm so sick of corned-beef hash that's all hash and no beef.'

Her mother tugged on the loose waistband of her home-sewn skirt. 'I'm not complaining. At my age, you're glad of keeping your figure by any means. I reckon I look like a young girl – from the back!' She laughed and primped her hair, though it was all stuffed under a scarf, as usual, but for a few stray steel-coloured strands. Her tired-looking face creased up around the eyes and at the sides of her mouth.

For the first time in a long time, Kitty studied her mother carefully. Though she'd recovered from her life-threatening chest infection, she looked gaunt and harried. Losing her job, moving to a slum and taking the notoriously slovenly, demanding and unpredictable Bert Longthorne back had all taken their toll on her beloved mam. 'You need a holiday,' Kitty said, an idea suddenly forming. 'Blackpool. Me and you. How about it? Just a weekend by the sea. Fish and chips and a night of dancing at the Winter Gardens. What do you say?'

Her mother looked at her quizzically. 'How on earth would we find the money for that, you daft ha'peth? And how could I leave your dad?'

Rolling her eyes, Kitty couldn't believe the change in her mother. 'A few months ago, you were working at Ford building engines! You had your own place, brought home a decent wage. Didn't you put money away?'

Her mother looked sheepishly down at her worn carpet slippers.

'Oh. I see,' Kitty said, withdrawing her arm from the crook of her mother's and stuffing her hands into her skirt pockets. 'He's gambled it all away, hasn't he? Or drunk it.'

'I know you don't understand why I took him back . . .'

'I do. He saved your life with that penicillin and never let you forget that for a second. He's not stupid, is he? You got back on your feet while he was inside, but the minute he's out, you've just slid back into being his servant.'

Her mother's tone was suddenly bitter. 'Look around you! All these women in this queue have had to give up good jobs so they can start washing their husbands' and sons' underpants and vests again. Beryl, over there, drove an ambulance 'til three weeks ago! She never had so much as a pushbike before the war. Alice – I haven't seen Alice Wregglesworth in anything but a pair of slacks since 1940 when she started on the buses as a mechanic. Look at her now in that dress and pinny. The most excitement she sees now that her Dennis is back is red-raddling her front step and going to the bingo to get away from his moods. We're not all lucky enough to be like you, young lady. I wanted better for you, and you're getting the career I'd always dreamed of with the chance of marrying well. But the rest of us – don't be so quick to judge, love. This is a man's world and women like me have to settle.'

'I promise I'm going to take you away for the weekend to Blackpool,' Kitty said, taking her mother's hand into hers. She thought about her grandmother's Whitby jet brooch that was the only thing of value she'd ever been given, passed onto her by her mother as a gift for securing a place as a junior nurse. Might Violet buy it from her? I'll find the money. And whatever happens with the election result, I'm going to make sure you've got somewhere better to live before the summer's out. One of the doctors at the hospital is looking for a housekeeper.'

'I'm grateful for the bit of work you got me in the hospital laundry, love. It keeps the wolf from the door, though I can't say getting up at four in the morning to travel all that way is much cop.'

'Exactly,' Kitty said, watching three women emerge from the shop with their baskets containing only a bacon parcel, flour and a rare tin of peaches that had been shipped from the other side of the world. It must have been somebody's birthday because Kitty reasoned that must have surely used up an entire month's tinned goods coupons! 'This house-keeping job would be out in Urmston. It's a children's doctor. He's very nice and has a young family, but his wife needs help. There's accommodation comes with the job. Posh, like.' Should she break the news to her mother that a convicted burglar and feckless layabout husband wouldn't be welcomed? Perhaps she could lure her mother to a job interview and let her see for herself the luxurious surrounds she could be living in, breathing the fresh air of Urmston instead of choking on the grim smog of Chorlton-on-Medlock. Then, perhaps, she'd be persuaded to give Kitty's errant father the heave-ho, once and for all. Might discovering Ned's survival and the extent of his injuries help her mother to change her priorities? Kitty said a silent prayer that Labour would get in. The wager with Ned was riding on it.

Chapter 16

Having helped her mother back to the semi-derelict house with the groceries, where her father was noticeable by his absence – no doubt propping up the bar in a stinking pub or playing cards in a back parlour somewhere – Kitty repaired to the nurses' home to snatch forty winks before she had to start her new night shift.

Perplexed by the sound of *Woman's Hour* wafting through the hallway, Kitty was surprised to find Matron in her study, listening to the wireless with the door open. Padding closer, Kitty wondered if there had been news about the election, but there was only speculation from a presenter who sounded rather like royalty. She was clearly a devotee of Churchill.

'Ah, Kitty!' Matron said, beckoning her to enter. 'Do come in. Sit! Sit!'

Swallowing hard, Kitty wondered if she was in trouble. Had Matron somehow found out about Ned? Was it possible she wasn't happy with Kitty's mother working in the laundry? Yet, she'd used Kitty's first name, rather than barking her surname, as usual. Tentatively, Kitty took a seat by the formidable head of the nursing staff.

'Why aren't you asleep, girl? You start the night shift tonight, don't you?'

'I have to look after my mother, matron. Help her with the shopping and a trip to the wash-house and that. She's living in a right dump. I've got to find her new digs. Anyway, I'm not sleeping very well at the moment, what with the heat.'

She considered the sleepless nights she'd spent, staring at the dancing streetlights on the ceiling that crept in through the crack in her curtains. In a bucolic scene involving sunlit fields and sheep – perhaps in the Lake District or the Peaks – she'd conjured an image of James going down on one knee and proposing to nursing's answer to Rita Heyworth. Violet had known her dowdy friend Kitty was hopelessly in love with the young doctor and that, against all social odds, they had begun to date. Yet it hadn't stopped Violet gunning for him herself. It had been as if Kitty's romantic aspirations weren't real or relevant. Though she acknowledged that Violet, with her flame-red locks and her nicely turned ankles and her middle-class upbringing, was undoubtedly the better catch for a doctor, it was the blatant disregard for her feelings that had kept Kitty awake of late, night after night. Violet had no conscience. And how much of Kitty's personal business had her so-called friend relayed to James? He'd been so cold with her ever since the night her father had reappeared on the scene. Was it possible that Violet had been dripping poison about her in the ear of the man she stupidly still loved?

Matron didn't need to hear about her secret suffering, however. 'I'll have a snooze this afternoon,' she said dismissively with a cheery smile. 'Anyway, I thought you'd be in the staffroom, if anywhere.'

Matron scoffed. 'I don't think I can bear another minute of Professor Baird-Murray's bleating on about a Tory victory, and how bad the Welfare State would be for the nation. Can you? All those men with their cigars, congratulating themselves on being masters of the universe!'

Smiling shyly, Kitty placed her hands in her lap and bit her lip. 'I suppose so.' She felt the heat in her cheeks, reluctant to betray her own political leanings, lest she said the wrong thing and was met with a cool reception. Tensions were running high in the hospital and the delay in announcing the result was only making matters worse. 'Are you in favour of a National Health Service, matron?'

Matron frowned. 'Good Lord, girl!' The sharp tone of her voice and startled look on her face couldn't be good news.

'I'm sorry, I didn't mean to—'

'Of course I'm in favour of a National Health Service! Let me tell you a story . . .' Matron poured Kitty a cup of tea from a china teapot. 'You might assume that everyone on the senior staff at Park Hospital was born with a silver spoon in their mouth.' She sipped from her own cup and daintily took a bite from a piece of shortbread. 'Let me tell you, Kitty Longthorne, I am the daughter of a market trader.'

'Never!'

'Yes. I absolutely am. My father fought in the Great War and was killed by the Hun, but before that, he ran a stall on Bury Market, selling black pudding.'

'Ooh, I love a nice black pudding, me.'

'He was the fifth son of a farmer, with no head for learning, no flair for managing livestock or the land. Nowt.' Suddenly, Matron sounded like a local woman, rather than the well-heeled, stuffy school-ma'am type Kitty had taken her for. 'Always the last one to make a bob, was my dad. But we scraped by, thanks to the black puddings he made from my granddad's pigs.'

'Fancy that!'

'There was many a winter when we had to burn the furniture we owned to keep warm. My mam chopped up a piano and threw that onto the fire during a rough spell.' Her sharp eyes suddenly seemed to swim with sorrow as she took this trip down memory lane. 'The war claimed Dad, the harsh winter of 1916 claimed my youngest brother, and my dear old Mam followed not long after with a terrible bladder infection. She should have seen a doctor, but she couldn't spare the fee.'

'I'm very sorry to hear it.'

'Thank you, Kitty. She was only in her fifties. I'm all that's left of my family.' The stalwart Matron dabbed at her eyes with a pristine white handkerchief. She cleared her throat and shook her head. 'So, in short, I have absolutely no doubt that this country is desperate for a Welfare State and a National Health Service. It's all very well if you're a toff like some of the consultants, here, and even some of your fellow nurses, but there's not much joy in living in a land where the rich get richer and the poor get poorer. It's not right. It's not Christian. A lot of wealthier folk have lost sight of that.'

Kitty looked at Matron open-mouthed, utterly taken aback that her superior should have been so frank and so overtly political. *Now*, she understood why Matron had been supportive of her, the night that her father had shown up at the nurses' home.

Unable to sleep and reflecting on what Matron had said about being Christian-minded, Kitty changed into her uniform and went over to the hospital before her shift started. Instead of making for the staffroom, she made her way to the ward and took a seat by the bedside of the girl who had had the backstreet abortion – Betty Buchanan. The girl was sleeping fitfully, but when she woke, she turned to Kitty with a look of alarm on her pale face.

'Nurse! Have you been there long?' She shuffled up the bed, grimacing with discomfort.

Kitty plumped her pillows and offered her a drink of water. 'Oh, not long at all.'

'Is something the matter?'

'Not at all. The doctors are pleased with your progress. I just thought I'd check on you.'

'Oh, that's kind. I haven't had any visitors since I come in.'

'Not even your family?' Kitty tried to imagine the scenario in which the girl might be abandoned by her parents in her hour of need.

Betty shook her head and looked ruefully into her glass of water.

'Would you like to talk about it?'

'I'm fine,' Betty said. But the dimpling in her chin said she was anything but.

Kitty held her hand. 'Go on. A trouble shared is a trouble halved. I won't breathe a word, I swear, if you want to talk.'

Her young patient dabbed at her eyes. 'They blame me, my family. They're ashamed. Everybody now knows Betty Buchanan got knocked up out of wedlock to a married man twice her age. But it weren't my fault! I didn't ask for it.'

'How do you mean?'

'This feller. A neighbour. He forced himself on me after the VE day celebrations. I was too embarrassed to tell anyone. Even Mam and Dad. Especially Mam and Dad. They're very religious, see. Dad had been a lay preacher when he was serving overseas. When my time of the month didn't turn up . . .'

What could Kitty possibly say to such a young girl who had been left to fend for herself in the direst of circumstances? She opened and closed her mouth but was lost for words.

'My dad threw money at me and told me to get rid.' When she spoke, her tone was utterly matter of fact, though Kitty reasoned that perhaps the girl had been left numb by the experience or else was still in shock. 'That's the last I seen of either of them.'

'Who called for a doctor?' Kitty asked.

Betty shrugged. 'One minute, I was lying on this woman's kitchen table. I'd had a full bottle of gin already.' She looked sheepish. 'You know what people say about gin and a hot bath?'

Kitty nodded, patting the girl's hand. 'Mothers' ruin. I think that's an old wives' tale, chuck.'

'Don't I know it? Anyway, I felt sick as a dog as it was, but then the woman knocked me out with ether on a rag or summat. Next minute, I'm lying under the bright lights of the operating theatre in here, being stitched up. No idea how I got here, but I was beside myself, thinking about how much it would all cost me and whether my mam would even wonder why I'd gone missing.' A solitary tear leaked onto her cheek.

'I . . .' Kitty searched for some advice she could give the girl but found none. 'Could you not have gone to the police about the neighbour?'

Betty shook her head. 'My word against his, isn't it? He's a well-respected family man who came home with a medal for bravery. I'm just – nothing. I've got no baby. I've got no home.'

'We'll find you somewhere to go, once you're ready to be discharged,' Kitty said, wondering if there was anything the hospital *could* do for cases like Betty's or the plights of the battered wives who'd been in the adjacent beds only days earlier. She'd have to make enquiries with Sister Iris or Matron. Perhaps the almoners could help.

Just as Kitty was thinking that the end of the war and the return of civilian patients to the hospital had thrown up a whole new raft of problems, Violet came running into the ward, red in the face and looking flustered. She was still dressed to assist in the operating theatre, as though she'd abandoned a patient, mid-surgery, having heard something dreadful that required immediate dissemination.

'Aye-aye,' Kitty said, getting to her feet and walking the length of the ward to meet her. 'What's all this, Vi? What's wrong?'

Violet came to a standstill, peering round at the patients and the other nursing staff, as though she was waiting for all eyes to be on her. 'Haven't you heard?' she asked. 'The results are in. You won't believe it. My father's going to be devastated.'

Sister Iris drew close. 'Well? Spit it out, girl! Which way did the wind blow?'

'Labour. Attlee's the new prime minister. And it wasn't a narrow victory either.' Violet sounded breathless. She clutched at her chest. 'They won by a landslide.'

Chapter 17

Two weeks later and Park Hospital was still buzzing with the news that Churchill's Tory Party had been defeated by Labour. During every moment snatched at break and meal times, the senior staff debated how the new government would affect the running of the hospital and the people in it. The junior staff were careful to keep their opinions to themselves. It wouldn't do to rattle the cage of Professor Baird-Murray or his acolytes.

Kitty was content to rejoice in private, however. After a war that had brought poverty, shame, sickness and huge loss to her family, she felt hopeful for the first time since she had begun her nursing training. Change was afoot, and it *had* to be for the better. James was noticeably more chipper, extolling the virtues of a National Health Service where care would be free for all. He didn't even seem perturbed by Violet's sulking and complaints that her father's taxes would fund the feckless among the working classes.

Fortunately, Violet had been only too happy to cheer herself up by buying Kitty's jet brooch. She'd gasped at the sight of the intricately carved woman's head and shoulders. The brooch had been intended to be worn during a period of mourning but now it was just a coveted item of jewellery.

'Oh, Kitty! What a dark horse you are. How funny that *you* should be sitting on a beautiful piece like this!'

Unsurprisingly, she'd haggled Kitty down until they'd agreed a price that was a fraction of its pre-war value. Money was money, however, and what Violet handed over for the brooch felt like a king's ransom, compared to the £2, 10 shillings per month that Kitty earned. It was certainly enough to quell the guilt at having parted with her only heirloom.

Using the money to book a weekend in Blackpool at the end of August for herself and her mother, as she'd promised, Kitty packed a small case, containing her scant supply of 'best' clothes. She met her mother in Manchester at the queue for the charabanc.

'Ooh, eh, our Kitty. I'm glad you talked me into this. This is right exciting!' her mother said, looking younger than she had done in a very long while, with her hair nicely styled and without a pinny to hide her dainty figure. Her mother clasped her hand and kissed her cheek with such exuberance, Kitty almost stumbled backwards. 'I left your dad with a sink full of dirty pots and told him to take a powder when he asked me to make his dinner before I left. You should have seen the poor soul. He had a face like a wet weekend in Scunthorpe!'

'As long as it wasn't a wet weekend in Blackpool!' Kitty giggled, squeezing her mother's hand. 'Anyway, this is our special girls' time. I got special leave from matron. I explained how we'd not had a proper holiday since 1933, when me and Ned were twelve and we went to Wales.'

Her mother sniffed hard at the mention of Ned. Blinking tears away, she looked up at the gleaming windows of the charabanc. 'She's a good'un, that matron, isn't she? You're lucky to have a champion like her, our Kitty. I can't believe she lent you the money for this. What a saint!' There was a wobble to her voice.

Kitty pushed down the rising tide of shame at this latest lie she'd felt compelled to tell. But truth was a luxury she couldn't afford, when her vulnerable mother's sensibilities were at stake. Knowing the brooch had been sold would break her heart. In any case, Kitty knew she'd made the right decision in whisking her mother away for a couple of days. She knew it would be a life-changing trip.

The charabanc was full of jolly holidaymakers, their spirits undampened by the light drizzle or smell of diesel that pervaded the coach or the bumpy ride as they made their pilgrimage to the north-west's favourite seaside town. Blackpool had enjoyed a boom-time during the war with so many GIs stationed nearby, flooding onto the Golden Mile with cash burning a hole in their uniform pockets, and with many a star-studded production from London being staged at the Grand Theatre. Yet many of the charabanc's travellers shared stories of not having been out of the city for years, though some had had children living nearby as evacuees.

A while into the journey, as the charabanc trundled into the vivid green of the Lancashire countryside, everybody joined in a singalong, bellowing their favourite Glen Miller and Vera Lynn numbers at the tops of their voices. By the time the famous metal spire of Blackpool Tower came into view, along with the thin, silver seam of the Irish Sea, Kitty delighted in her mother solemnly warbling that there would 'Always be an England', along with the other teary-eyed passengers. It felt good to be drawing a line under the war and dark times. Could this trip be the turning point for the Longthornes?

*

When she stepped off the coach, glad to breathe in the fresh air instead of the stink of the charabanc's engine, the wind whipped at Kitty's cheeks, bringing with it the smell of brine from the sea and hot fat from some chippy on the Golden Mile. Her mouth watered and her stomach rumbled audibly.

'Let's get to our digs,' she said, waiting in line to lug their cardboard cases from the baggage compartment. 'I booked us a lovely B & B with a sea view.'

'A sea view!' Her mother's face lit up. 'Good Lord, what have I done to deserve a girl like you?' She grabbed Kitty and planted a kiss on her cheek. 'You're a little belter, what are you?'

Already, there was colour in her mother's normally pasty cheeks as she buttoned up her jacket against the wind and smiled at the sight of the sea – some way out beyond the brown rippled sand, thanks to a low tide. The tinny strains of merry-go-round music and the laughter of other holidaymakers wafted towards them both. Her mother giggled. The frivolity was catching!

'I always loved Blackpool when I was a little girl,' she told Kitty. 'Your gran and granddad used to bring me here on my birthday. Dad told me it was just like Paris, thanks to the tower, but with better grub and prettier girls! We were always lucky with the weather. It was usually scorching hot, even though it was only mid-June. Like the sun was shining just for me!'

Kitty smiled, glad that her mother was remembering better times. This was exactly what she hoped for – she wanted her mother to remember life before Bert Longthorne, with his domestic dictatorship and drunken deviousness. Perhaps Elsie Longthorne could be persuaded yet again that she was strong enough to be alone; that her priority was not to be a drudge for, and a slave to, the whim of a weak and manipulative man.

The Golden Mile was a dizzying whirl of noise and spectacle, shining with the brilliance of a thousand bulbs. Its shops, selling Blackpool rock and ice cream, and its stalls, peddling sweet treats, sideshows and postcards, stretched along the busy main boulevard.

'Look at that beach!' Kitty said, pointing to the mass of occupied deckchairs that rendered the brown sands almost invisible. 'All them men with knotted hankies on their heads. I remember that from when we came with our Ned!'

'Don't they look daft?' Her mother laughed out loud, walking with a spring in her step and swinging her suitcase. 'My old dad did that, and all. He used to roll his trousers up, too. I wonder what the Yanks make of us.'

'Probably think we're barmy. Come on, Mam! Let's stop for some fish and chips on the way. I'm ravenous.'

Slowly and with full stomachs, they meandered their way to the guesthouse, which proved to be basic but clean and comfortable, with a breathtaking view of the length of the seafront. Having unpacked, Kitty suggested they go for another walk.

'If you don't mind, love, I might have forty winks,' her mother said, rubbing her feet as she sat on her single bed. 'I don't normally get the chance. If I'm not working, your dad's asking me to do this or fetch that for him, the lazy beggar.'

Kitty checked her watch and frowned. They only had a limited amount of time in Blackpool and she wanted to make it count. 'Go on, then. Half an hour, and then I'll have to get you up, Mam, because I've booked us tickets to a show.'

'Which show?'

'It's a surprise.'

Her mother nodded, her eyelids already starting to droop. 'Just a quick snooze. Then I'm all yours.'

Staring out of the guesthouse window, Kitty considered what she had planned for her mother. She felt a pang of guilt at the lie she'd just told, but hopefully her mother wouldn't hold it against her when she discovered the real surprise that Kitty had up her sleeve.

Chapter 18

An hour later, they were back on the promenade, making their way into the fray of day trippers and holidaymakers; watching the trams rattle up and down the seafront. Regularly glancing at her wristwatch, Kitty led them briskly up a side street to a dank-looking café. Through the greasy window, it was clear that the place was empty, but for an elderly couple, looking utterly glum and not speaking.

Her mother pulled her back. 'Why are we going in here? I want to stay where I can see the sea.' She glanced down the street. 'I can't see it from here.'

'Mam. Please. We've got to go in here. Trust me. It's part of my plans for you.'

'Plans for me?' She narrowed her eyes.

'You'll see.'

Inside, Kitty ushered her mother to a table in the corner. The place smelled of stale lard with a top-note of wet dog, but it didn't matter. It was quiet and off the beaten track. It was exactly what the situation demanded.

'Couldn't we have gone to the Kardomah? It's years since I had a coffee there. Your dad took me there once or twice when we started courting.'

'Cup of tea, Mam?' Kitty left her mother seated at a table for four and approached the counter. It wasn't the sort of place that had waitress service.

The café owner was a large woman, wearing an apron that

had once been white. She wore her grey hair beneath a pink hairnet and had a sizeable wart on her chin that sprouted hairs. Kitty balked, but none of that mattered.

'Two teas, please.'

The woman poured treacly looking tea from a large metal catering teapot into two cheap porcelain cups. As she did so, the door to the café tinkled and out of the corner of her eye, Kitty saw a man enter. Her pulse quickened as the man paused in the middle of the room, looking in her mother's direction.

'Make that three teas,' Kitty said.

She turned around and locked eyes with the new customer. They exchanged a knowing nod. So far, her mother hadn't looked up from the menu she was studying. The man approached the counter and took two of the teas, ignoring the café owner's look of alarm as she caught sight of his face at close quarters.

'You made it,' Kitty whispered.

'I got here yesterday. I haven't slept a wink.'

'Come on, then.'

Together they made their way to the table. Finally, her mother looked up.

'Ooh, hey! Who's this?' she asked Kitty. It was clear from her voice that she was startled by the sudden appearance of the strange man with his makeshift nose and ruined features. She visibly shrank from him and clasped her handbag close against her body. 'Is this one of your patients?' Then she seemed to take in the detail of the side of his face that was perfect. Her eyes widened. She gasped. 'Ned?'

When she stood up abruptly, the table shook, spilling the tea into the saucers.

'Are you all right, Mrs?' the elderly gentleman at the only other occupied table asked.

For a few heartbeats, she stared in silence. Then a smile slowly warmed her pale face. 'I'm better than all right,' Kitty's mother said, never taking her eyes off Ned's face.

She flung her arms around her long-lost son, tears rolling onto her cheeks. If Ned's burns still smarted, it didn't show. He enfolded her in a tight embrace, snuggling his damaged face into her neck.

'Mam! Oh, Mam. I've missed you so much.'

Kitty watched as the tears from Ned's good eye splashed onto her mother's shoulder. She put her arms around each of them so that they became a huddle of love, wonder and relief.

'It's been years and we've heard next to nowt,' her mother said. She hiccupped as she spoke. 'I-I thought my boy was dead and gone for the longest time. Then we got this telegram, saying you were in a Japanese prisoner-of-war camp.' She took a battered piece of paper from her hard-framed handbag and unfolded it with some reverence. It was the telegram. Her finely plucked eyebrows sunk low above her watery eyes. 'But the Japanese haven't surrendered yet and none of our lads have made it home. So, how is it you're sat here?'

They took a seat at the table, Ned facing his mother and Kitty, while Kitty put her arm around the quaking shoulders of a woman who looked like she'd seen a ghost, only to find he was still breathing.

'It's a long story, Mam.' Ned looked sheepishly at his cup and tea-filled saucer. He started to mop the spillage up, holding a paper serviette in his trembling hand.

'I've got all weekend, son. Out with it.' Their mother reached over and stroked his malformed nose. When he shrank from her touch, she settled for holding his hand. 'Where's my handsome boy gone? Oh, Ned. What on God's earth happened to you? Tell your mam.'

Ned inhaled deeply and puffed the air out slowly. 'I'm not sure I can talk about it.'

'You've been away for years without so much as a letter. Try.'

He squeezed his good eye shut, though his new glass eye stared blankly ahead. 'I saw some terrible things while I was in the Far East. Thousands died. Tens of thousands. We surrendered in Hong Kong and . . . I ended up being herded with a bunch of other lads from my battalion to work on the Burma railway. They worked us like beasts of burden, the Japanese did. We weren't fed properly. Just rice and the odd bit of veg. Hardly any clean water. We were starving but we had to build this blinking railway, hacking our way through thick Siamese jungle in torrential rain. It was a nightmare. The dysentery and other diseases . . . ulcers that stripped a man's flesh right down to the bone. Brutal beatings for looking at a Japanese soldier the wrong way. I'd never seen the likes of it in my life.'

'You were a slip of a boy when you ran off to enlist! Course you'd never seen the flaming likes. What life had *you* had?' There was a ruefulness to her mother's voice. She released her grip on his hand.

'Anyway . . .' Ned slurped at his cup, catching the dribbles with a second serviette. 'God must have been watching over me, because I stayed strong. Even though I was nowt more than a walking skeleton, I didn't fall ill. Most of my friends were dead after a couple of months.' He looked down at his scarred hands and sighed. 'Anyway, the Japs decided they needed workers on their docks. So, me and some Yanks were marched all the way back to Japan.'

'You marched from Siam to Japan? No wonder you've been gone years.'

'That's the least of it,' Ned said. 'I got these burns on the last leg of the journey home.'

'He got torpedoed on a supply ship, didn't you, our Ned?' Kitty offered.

'Aye. Me and some of the Yankee fellers escaped from our prisoner-of-war camp. We watched a mate get beaten to death. He got caught having a bit of a chuckle at one of their officers – a right nasty little bleeder, who slipped on some mud and fell on his arse at roll call. Next minute, there's this big one with a massive bit of bamboo and he's . . .' He looked at his mother and shook his head. 'It doesn't matter. But we'd had enough, me and some of the Yankee lads. We made a pact to get out – and we did! It took us months, but we walked all the way from Japan.'

'I don't believe you,' his mother said. 'How the hell can you *walk* back to Manchester from Japan? You'd stick out like a sore thumb, for a start, with all them Orientals.'

'We didn't walk to flipping Manchester, Mam. Come on! But we did walk right through Asia. All right?' Ned avoided her gaze. 'Well – we might have stolen some horses or the odd bicycle to cover a few miles, but that doesn't matter. You're living on your wits when you're on the run. You've got to do what you've got to do, haven't you? Anything's better than staying in one of them camps 'til it's your turn to die. Anyway, eventually, when we got further west, we bumped into some allies.' He treated them both to a crooked smile. 'I nearly copped a bullet then! They thought we were spies or summat. They took some persuading, that's for sure. But, turns out, my mate Dwight came from the same town as one of them. He squared it all. That's when we got a lift on a Red Cross supply ship across the Indian Ocean.'

Kitty's mother laced her fingers together and sat up straight in her chair. 'And when was that, exactly? Because those burns have healed up nicely and you're no skeleton now. But that *wasn't* the nose you were born with. Even I can tell it's not just scar tissue. Some doctor's had you under his knife. Where have you been since you got torpedoed, son?' She grabbed Ned's chin and angled his face towards her so that he had no option but to look her directly in the eye. 'You're only giving me half the truth, young man.'

'Jesus, Mam!' Ned said, pulling away. 'Can't you just be happy that I'm alive and I'm back? All I want to do is get through my surgeries and try to make a normal life for myself. I've been to hell and survived to tell the tale.'

'And me, Kitty and your dad haven't been living a waking nightmare? Wondering what had become of you?'

'I'm sorry. I didn't want to burden you with my—'

'Your what?'

Ned closed his good eye. 'Problem.'

'Aye-aye. Here we go,' Kitty's mother said, nudging Kitty and faking a smile. Then her face crumpled into a frown. 'Let me guess. Money. It's always flaming money with the Longthorne men. And there's me, thinking my troubles were finally over!'

PART II

—

1947

Chapter 19

'Do us a favour, love,' Kitty's father said, pausing only to belch loudly and thump himself in the chest. 'Get us another slice of bread and marg off your mam.' He rubbed his belly and held the side plate out expectantly.

Standing over him, imagining wiping a piece of bread all over his stubbled face, smothered in the foul-tasting margarine that her mother insisted on using in these times of stringent rationing, Kitty smiled wryly. 'No.'

'No?'

'You heard. Mam's having to make everything go a bit further, now Ned's home.' She looked over at her brother, who was sitting by the fire, shivering, though he was dressed in three jumpers and an overcoat. The flames licked half-heartedly around the coals. 'You get what you're given. Mam might not tell you that, but I don't care if I do.'

Her father scowled at her, dragging the newspaper out from under the seat pad of his armchair and sitting back down. With a dirty fingernail, he jabbed at the photo of the frozen scene beneath the headline. 'Worst winter on record,' he simply said, as if this excused his demands. 'When there's twenty-foot snowdrifts out there, I want feeding. How else is a man to keep warm?'

'Maybe by getting off your jacksy and finding a job, Dad. How about that? Even our Ned's got work since his treatment finished.'

'Even our Ned. Thanks, Kitty,' Ned said, stoking the fire to no effect. 'Crikey, it's freezing in here. Haven't we got anything else we can burn?' He looked around the room. His good eye fell on an old gramophone that Kitty's mother had bought in a jumble sale.

'Put more coal on the fire, Elsie!' Bert yelled through to the kitchen, grabbing the poker from Ned. 'This is all bloody stones!'

Finally, Kitty's mother appeared in the doorway of the lounge. 'Not on your Nelly, Bert Longthorne. That bag cost me four shillings and ten pence. It's got to last and all, unless you're sat on some winnings you forgot to tell me about.'

Kitty's father grumbled and settled back into his old chair, folding his arms tightly around his chest. 'Fat flaming chance. Fred and the lads won't come and play cards now we're in this dump. How can I set up a game with no back parlour?'

But Kitty's mother had disappeared again.

Kitty followed her into the kitchen, beating a retreat to the warmth of the big black range that made the tiny place the only comfortable space during the infernal freezing cold. Helping her mother to dish up the sausages and instant mash, made from powdered potato, at a time when potatoes were incredibly scarce, she thought about how the end of the war had offered everyone such hope for a bright new beginning. Yet here her mother was, two years on, scratching a Sunday dinner together from substandard ingredients for a family that was falling apart at its seams; her face, a picture of prematurely ageing misery and malnutrition.

'This looks smashing, Mam. I don't know how you manage it,' Kitty said, arranging the grey sausages, which were mainly stuffed with rusk and fat, on the plates. 'A meal fit for a king!'

'Oh, go away!' her mother said, smiling. She suddenly shuffled closer to Kitty and whispered secretively in her ear. 'Minnie, next door, said her Tom can get his hands on some knock-off meat. Lamb. Half a lamb, Kitty! Imagine that!'

Kitty frowned. 'I know times are hard. None of us expected this winter or rationing getting stricter. I'm as fed up as you. I doubt I'll get back to Davyhulme before the end of the week if it doesn't pack it in snowing! But don't you think it would be better for Dad to get a job and earn an honest crust than getting knock-off meat from her next door?'

'Our Ned's promised her a couple of raincoats in lieu.'

'He's stealing? From the factory?'

Her mother shushed her. 'We've got to eat, Kitty, love. We're not all lucky enough to get meals and lodging with our jobs like you. Just be glad you get three square meals a day.'

'You'll get turfed out of this new flat if the coppers catch you, Mam.'

'Salford Brow is hardly Buckingham Palace, love.'

Kitty could feel irritation itch away at the base of her neck. 'No, but at a time when the housing shortage is getting worse, not better, just thank your lucky stars that James pulled some strings with his dad's mates in Salford council, and got you bumped up the list for a place.' There was a flicker of warmth in her chest at the thought of James coming to her family's aid, yet again. Then she thought of Violet, and the flicker died.

'I'd sooner have one of the maisonettes. We're rammed in here like sardines. The cockroaches are a blinking pain in the neck.'

'There're fewer of them than in that hovel in Chorlton-on-Medlock. And there's an indoor toilet! Count your blessings, Mam.'

Her mother's lips thinned to a line. 'We should call you Sister Kitty, not Nurse Kitty. The nuns have got nothing on you. Or maybe we'll just promote you to Saint Kitty. Yes, I know what you did for us. I just can't get used to being in a flat, is all. Or so far from Hulme. It's not the same people around here. It's not my people.'

'You've got a steady job as a machinist, Mam, and a decent roof over your head. Just don't risk any of this for a couple of roast dinners. Thieving is thieving. I thought you were honest as the day's long. Remember what you swore to Ned in Blackpool, if he got involved in any funny business back in Manchester? You allowed him home on the condition that he kept his nose clean. He was damned lucky that the feller he owed money to got killed in Dunkirk. Don't you realise, it's nothing short of a miracle that he's got away with impersonating a dead Yankee airman; getting free treatment under false pretences? I had to *beg* James to file that report to keep him out of military prison. Saying our Ned got amnesia from the explosion and didn't know up from down, let alone remember who he was. James could lose his job for telling lies like that!'

'He is a good feller, that doctor of yours.'

Kitty chewed her lip and frowned. 'He's not my doctor. Anyway. Never mind that. Our Ned's been given a second chance, along with his new face and a clean slate. So, why's the ungrateful beggar back to his old ways? Because he's a chip off the old Bert Longthorne block, that's why! You shouldn't encourage him, Mam!'

'Go easy on your brother,' her mother said, putting two

sprouts on each plate. 'He's got a mountain to climb with that face of his. What girl's going to marry our Ned? What firm is going to give him a well-paid job? People are cruel, even when it's a war hero. I was lucky to get him in at Bergman's. As it happens, the boss was a Japanese prisoner of war too. He felt sorry for our Ned.'

Their conversation was interrupted, however, by her father stomping into the kitchen. He looked down at the meagre serving of grey, drab food on the old chipped china plates that had belonged to Kitty's grandmother.

'This tripe *again*? You're not on, Elsie! I'm not having that.' He picked up the plate full of food and threw it into the embers of the range's oven. 'I've had it with this! I'm off to the pub. I'll get pie and chips there.'

'We can't afford it, Bert! Wait! Have mine!'

Her mother followed her father to the front door, pleading with him as he paused by the fireplace to grab some money out of the bills jar, stuffing it into his coat pocket. She watched as he lumbered off along the landing to the stairwell without so much as a backwards glance.

The February snow was still falling in earnest. An Arctic wind blew into the flat.

Kitty gently moved her weeping mother aside and closed the door. 'Come on, Mam. Don't let your dinner go cold.'

Ned approached and, together, they held their mother until her tears stopped falling.

Gently, she pushed them both away, collecting their plates from the tiny kitchen table and holding them out. The gravy was beginning to congeal. 'Here! Don't let this go to waste!'

Sitting with their dinner on their laps in the lounge, they ate in mournful silence. Outside, it looked like God had torn a celestial eiderdown and was shaking the white feathers onto the earth below. Kitty's thoughts turned to making beds on the wards and she started to worry that she would get the sack if she didn't get back to the hospital in time for the night shift.

'I'm going to have to make tracks, Mam,' she said when she'd finished eating the bland meal. She put her cutlery together and swiped Ned's plate from under his nose, just as he'd shovelled in his final mouthful, rising to take the crockery into the kitchen. 'This was lovely and I wish I could stay longer, but the wards are going to be overflowing in this snow. Matron's depending on me. I've got a junior nurse beneath me now. I'm showing her the ropes!'

Her mother stood, taking the plates from Kitty, her own stacked on top with half the dinner remaining uneaten. 'My girl, the teacher!' She smiled weakly. 'I'm sorry about before – calling you Saint Kitty and that. I didn't mean it. I am so, so proud of you, Kitty, love.' She hastened into the kitchen, setting the plates down with a thud, and suddenly burst into tears.

'Oh, Mam! Don't cry! Stuff him! Lock the dead-leg out. Let him go and find some other doormat to cook his tea and darn his socks.'

'I can't lock him out, you soft ha'peth! He'd freeze to death – or kick the door down, making a laughing stock of me in front of all the neighbours. And he saved my life. How could I? I'm stuck with him.' Her sobs grew louder.

Kitty embraced her mother, dearly wishing that she could one day earn enough to take her away from her father and these low-rent digs, to set her up in her own private house or flat. How much would a little two-up, two-down or a small cottage in a nice area like Urmston or Eccles even cost? More than she could ever afford, that was for certain!

'You don't owe him a shilling, Mam. I asked him to get that penicillin. He was just trying to curry favour to get back in your life. That's all it was.'

Her mother broke free of the embrace, suddenly quaking, though it was impossible to tell if that was from the biting cold or adrenalin from the quarrel with her father. 'He loves me.'

Frustrated, Kitty tutted and rolled her eyes. 'I'm not disputing that! But he knows how to get you over a barrel. Of course you were always going to take him back if he got you the medicine that saved your life. Bert Longthorne is a manipulator and a liar, Mam. He always has been. He's a lazy layabout and pollutes the good in this family. I would have nicked that penicillin myself, if you'd not made me swear otherwise.'

Their debate was brought to an abrupt end as the sound of splintering wood from the lounge made them both jump. Fearing her father was kicking the door down, Kitty ran through to find Ned breaking the gramophone's base into pieces and throwing the wood onto the fire. The horn lay decapitated on the hearth.

'Ned! What are you doing, you berk?' Kitty yelled.

'It's cold enough to freeze the balls on a brass monkey!' he said simply, stoking the rising flames that licked up the chimney. 'I couldn't bear it anymore.'

'Oh, you didn't!' her mother said. 'Ned! That was your grandmother's!'

'You told me you got it from a jumble.'

'It wasn't yours to burn, young man.' Her mother's shoulders slumped as she stared at the smouldering remains.

'What are we going to do, then? Freeze to death? You can't enjoy Glen Miller if you're stiff as a board in your armchair.' Ned picked up the horn. 'We can trade this for scrap once the snow's gone.'

'The apple didn't fall far from the tree, did it, Ned?' Kitty said sourly, putting her arm around her mother. 'Fencing stolen meat and ruining Mam's prized possessions? Think on! It's bad enough having one rotten apple in the barrel. If you touch anything else of Mam's without her permission, so help me God, I'll—'

Ned rounded on her, drawing close enough for her to see the tiny red capillaries James had painted in the corners of his glass eye. 'You'll what?'

Kitty pushed him hard in the shoulder, as she had done when they'd fought as children. 'I'll make you regret coming back from Japan.'

'You and whose army?' He pushed her back.

Balling her fist, the twelve-year-old inside her was ready to plant a punch squarely on Ned's jaw, but, then, she realised the war had already given Ned the battering of a lifetime. She beat him half-heartedly with her words instead. 'I'll make you wish they'd thrown you in the Mekong River and left you to rot, if you come the hurry-up like that again.'

Their mother finally drove the twins apart and Kitty left with a heavy heart to embark on the epic trek back to Davyhulme through the snow drifts.

As no buses were running down Bury New Road, she trudged the mile into Manchester city centre, skidding along in her second-hand sheepskin boots – hand-me-downs from Violet, the soles of which had been worn treacherously smooth and thin over time. Kitty had had to improvise new treads by binding the feet in a web of sturdy string, giving them just enough traction on the slippery pavements. As she passed Strangeways prison, she kept her hood up and her head down against the biting blizzard, barely glimpsing the ghostly bomb-ravaged remains of the once-glorious assize courts and the red-brick hulk of the prison beyond. By the time she'd skidded and stumbled her way past the cathedral to Deansgate, she was exhausted and out of breath.

As her mind swirled faster than the eddies of snow with thoughts of her mother's predicament and her brother's deteriorating behaviour, she failed to notice the tall man in the dark overcoat and trilby, emerging from the picture house. They collided, sending him skittering onto his bottom in the slush. Kitty yelped.

'Oh dear! I'm *so* sorry!' she said, extending her gloved hand to help him up.

'No! No! I beg *your* pardon, miss! It was entirely my fault. I should have been watching where I was going. What an oaf I am.'

The man took her hand and got to his feet. Though his voice was all too familiar, Kitty didn't recognise him until he was once again upright and their eyes met.

'Dr Collins!' she said, smiling at Park Hospital's young anaesthetist.

'Why! If it isn't the lovely Nurse Kitty!' He brushed the snow off his coat, blushing and beaming at her. 'It's only fitting that I should have fallen at your feet!' His neck reddened. 'I-I say, would you like to join me for a coffee?'

Kitty glanced at her watch. This chance encounter with Richard Collins felt like the start of something, but she was running late.

'Well?' he asked.

Chapter 20

'I think I'll just have a coffee made with milk,' Kitty said, smiling coyly at Richard as she took a seat opposite him at the only available table on the ground floor of the busy Market Street coffee house. She draped her soaking coat carefully over the back of her chair, feeling ungainly and utilitarian in a place that was otherwise filled with chic-looking women in furs and elegant men in Crombies. Other newcomers filed up the sleek, winding staircase to the galleried landing that was the second floor, as if they sought their rightful place above the lesser snow-sodden souls of Manchester. 'I haven't been to the Kardomah since . . .' She thought about the last date she'd had with James before the end of the war – when they'd gazed into each other's eyes and such promise had seemed to be in the air. No. Richard didn't need to know about that failure. 'It's a good long while, anyway.' She giggled nervously. 'I feel so out of place in these ridiculous boots! You must think me quite the washer-woman in all these layers.'

'Nonsense,' he said, setting his hat on the empty chair beside him and smoothing down his sandy-coloured hair. 'You're dressed for the weather. We're in the grip of a deep freeze that would give the Russians a run for their money! It's a good job I did bump into you. We wouldn't want you freezing to death on the way to the hospital. Walking all the way from Cheetham, indeed!'

He studied the menu. Kitty took the opportunity to steal a quick glance at the clock on the wall above them. It told her she'd better be quick, if she didn't want to incur Matron's wrath. She had half an hour before her bus departed. Stopping off for an impromptu coffee with a doctor she'd barely spoken to before with so little time spare seemed positively reckless. Right at that moment, though, the thought of thawing out with a hot drink trumped any fear of reprisal for being late – and, of course, she was terribly flattered to have been asked in the first place.

The waitress approached, wearing a black-and-white uniform. She looked expectantly at Richard who placed their orders for the delicious-smelling coffee.

'Cake?' he asked Kitty.

'Oh, I couldn't possibly!' Kitty thought about the meagre meal she'd failed to enjoy at her mother's. Her stomach growled, yet she didn't want to appear greedy.

'I insist!'

Before she could protest, he'd ordered them both a slice of marble cake.

Finally, they were alone in a place that smelled like heaven and that felt like another world, untouched by the war or rationing or the nation's continued collective suffering. Kitty found herself lost for words. Richard seemed to find words for them both, however.

'I've just been to see a matinee of *The Postman Always Rings Twice*,' he said. 'Have you seen it? It came out last year, and I've already seen it twice, but I'm such a fan of Lana Turner.' He grinned and blushed. 'Although, I have read the novel at least three times, so it's not entirely all about her.'

Kitty wracked her brains for something to contribute but only came up with, 'I haven't been to the pictures in an age. I just don't get enough time off, and when I do, I have to visit my family.'

'It's noir.'

'What's noir?' Kitty was puzzled. Was he commenting on her family obligations? Did he know something about the Longthornes? Was it a pointed comment about her father's criminal record? Or had he simply ignored every word she'd just said?

Richard laughed. '*The Postman Always Rings Twice*. It's classic noir. I love that kind of thing. I quite like French films too. *La Belle et la Bête*. That came out last autumn. I went to see it when I was in Paris. Have you been?'

'I'm afraid I haven't been further than the Eiffel Tower of the North.'

He looked at her blankly.

'Blackpool Tower,' she explained, hoping he'd see her joke.

He didn't. 'Paris in the autumn is magical,' he continued. 'The Rive Gauche, the Louvre, the Folies Bergère! No wonder Hitler was determined to take Paris by force. She really is a beauty.'

'Aren't French films and the Folies Bergère a bit . . . blue?'

He shook his head. 'There's nothing blue about taking an interest in our continental neighbours. I worked in a field hospital in Dieppe during the war. France is a wonderful place. I'm quite the Francophile, you know.'

Kitty was rapidly beginning to feel out of her depth. Paris. Noir films. Naked dancing ladies. How could she possibly hold her own with a man of such – *was* it even sophistication? 'And there was me, thinking you were an anaesthetist.'

Their cake and coffee arrived. For the next twenty minutes, Kitty's eyes were intermittently on the clock as she listened to this perfectly nice young doctor talk about his role in the war and his family who owned a country estate near the Welsh border and his intense interest in Cubism and Walter Gropius' Bauhaus school of architecture and design and French cheeses. At no point did he ask Kitty anything about herself, beyond whether she'd like to accompany him to see a film when the weather improved.

Kitty stared at him open-mouthed for a few moments until finally she rediscovered the power of her own voice. 'You're asking me on a date?'

Richard laughed dryly. 'Yes. Of course. If you'd like.' He blushed.

She liked the way he coloured up when he was embarrassed. She wondered if he had gabbled on so, purely because he'd been as taken aback by the chance meeting as she had and had been as nervous as she had. She was impressed when he paid the bill, helped her on with her damp coat and offered to drive them both back to Park Hospital in his new Hillman Minx.

'All right,' she said. 'Yes, I'd like that very much, Dr Collins.'

They drove slowly through the snow, leaving the stinking clouds of diesel fumes emitted by the buses and lorries far behind. Their route took them through the terraced slums of Salford, eventually heading south and out towards Davyhulme. The further they went, the deeper the snow became; the more insistent the downpour of fat flakes grew, shining like gold dust in the yellow street lights of a late afternoon. The roads became whiter and more difficult to navigate with the Hillman skidding periodically as Richard negotiated a stretch of ice.

'I've never seen anything like it,' he said, peering through the windscreen, past the frenetic windscreen wipers that were only just keeping up. They passed streets of terraced housing that were almost buried beneath a thick blanket of white. 'I really do worry for the poor souls living in those houses. Look! There's hardly a single chimney pot with smoke coming out of it.'

'That's because nobody can afford coal,' Kitty said. 'And when they can, it goes nowhere in this weather. It's full of stone.' She was tempted to tell him about Ned's desecration of her mother's precious gramophone but thought better of it. A doctor from wealthy landed gentry who studied architecture and fine foreign cheeses in his spare time perhaps wouldn't understand the plight of Elsie and Bert, with their nocturnal cockroaches and sausages made from breadcrumbs. Suddenly, she felt cheap and irrelevant, sitting in a car that would surely have cost the same as a humble two-bedroom house, wearing second-hand boots that were reinforced by parcel string. She was glad to be out of the snow, though.

They rode on in companionable silence that was punctuated only by Richard bursting into the odd bout of cheerful whistling and by the whine and growl of the engine. Finally, Park Hospital loomed before them, snow-covered and eerily luminous in the dark.

Richard deftly pulled the car into the carpark and came to a standstill. When he patted Kitty's hand, she didn't pull away.

'Shall I find you on your next evening off, then?' he asked, staring ahead through the windscreen.

Kitty bit her lip. 'Yes. Thanks for a . . . this afternoon was quite unexpected.' She flashed him with a bewildered smile. 'Thank you.'

As she got out of the car, she looked up at one of the windows on the upper floor to see James peering down at her. She hurried towards the nurses' home to change, grinning to herself - more tickled at being spotted getting out of another doctor's car by the man she'd loved than at the baffling turn of events that had driven her from a family argument straight into a snow-drenched date.

Chapter 21

Dressed in her nurse's uniform and ready for her shift, Kitty made her way over to the hospital, gazing at the windows to see if James might appear a second time. Her thoughts were interrupted by the approach of an ambulance, pulling up right in front of the entrance for emergency admissions.

The driver hopped out of the cab and opened the doors at the back. His colleague sprang out and, together, they lifted the invalid out on a trolley. Normally, Kitty would scurry past, leaving the care of the patient to the emergency nurses and doctors, but on this occasion, she balked at the sight of a woman whose head was covered in blood and who was clearly struggling to breathe.

'This one's critical, nurse,' one of the men said. He spoke rapidly. 'Bad head injury. Suspected broken rib and punctured lung. Severe blood loss and dehydration. They're run off their feet in there.' He nodded towards the brightly lit emergency department beyond the doors. 'I could do with your help right away.'

Nodding, Kitty remained absolutely calm and took a hold of the drip that had been hooked up to the woman.

'Don't worry love,' she said, though the woman was out cold. 'We'll get you fixed up in here.'

Once inside, Kitty locked eyes with the receptionist. She kept her voice strong but calm. 'Can we get a doctor to examine this woman immediately please?'

'We haven't got one spare at the moment,' the receptionist said.

Kitty looked at the woman's grey-tinged, mottled pallor and could see her chest barely rising and falling. 'We need to get her straight to theatre to get her lung seen to or this lady isn't going to make it,' she whispered urgently to the men, hoping that neither the sick and injured in the waiting room nor the patient herself would hear her.

The men nodded.

Realising that she was now late for her shift, but seeing that the emergency department was indeed woefully under-staffed, as nurses scurried from bed to bed, tending to patients that were dangerously close to having frozen to death or else were suffering frost bite, Kitty pushed thoughts of an angry Sister Iris from her mind. Prioritise. That was what the doctors did and that was what Kitty had to do. They wheeled the woman down the brightly lit corridor towards the operating theatre.

'What's the lady's name?' Kitty asked the ambulance man.

'Dora Mackie,' he said.

'Does she have relatives? Who knows she's here?'

'The neighbour raised the alarm. Thinks she'd been lying at the bottom of the stairs for hours. Apparently, her children were all crying – she's got five under the age of six, if you can believe it – and when the noise didn't pipe down by teatime, the neighbour realised something was up.'

'No father?'

The ambulance man shook his head. 'There was a wedding photo on the sideboard but no man at home when we were there.'

Kitty looked at Dora's battered face, seeing beyond the blood from her head wound. Her lip was split and her nose had been broken, by the looks. There was bruising on her cheekbone, close to her eye socket. 'I think there's more than meets the eye to this one. I reckon Mr Mackie's out there, drinking himself into a stupor in some pub so he can't feel the sting of the split skin on his knuckles.' She tutted and pressed her lips together in disapproval. 'We get plenty of women like this on the wards. The war has returned men that are unexploded bombs, waiting to go off.'

'I don't think it's fair to badmouth heroes,' the older of the ambulance men said, frowning at her. 'Men that have seen active service have got a lot on their plates when they get back. Feeding families and starting all over again. It's not easy, you know.'

Kitty could sense that she'd hit a raw nerve. Then she remembered she'd heard that one of the ambulance drivers – a man named Bob – had won a raft of medals for bravery in the navy, only to be demobbed and to find that his wife had upped sticks and moved in with his best friend. The staffroom was often abuzz with titbits of gossip like that. Perhaps this was Bob. She tried to glimpse his name badge, but they were walking too quickly along the corridor.

'That's no excuse for—'

'For what?' The ambulance man glared at her.

The words 'using women as punch-bags' died on Kitty's tongue, unsaid. They merely pushed on in uncomfortable silence.

Lying on her trolley, there was an ominous rattling in Dora's throat where she was failing to cough up the mucus gathering in her respiratory tract.

Kitty took her hand, feeling an untimely end was danger-ously close if her lung wasn't re-inflated. 'Nearly there, Dora. Don't worry. You'll be in good hands.'

They reached the operating theatre, pulling the trolley up just outside the doors. Kitty went on ahead, expecting to find the surgeons in the midst of scheduled procedures. Peering through the windows in the double doors of one of the theatres, she could see that Mr Fotherington-Smythe, the brain surgeon, was busy with a patient, surrounded by a small team of nursing staff and a junior doctor. He was wielding a scalpel with care and precision and there was no way she could disturb him.

Double doors in the adjacent theatre swung open suddenly and a trolley was wheeled out, bearing a woman whose neck was bandaged heavily.

Kitty poked her head inside, squinting at the bright overhead lights that bounced off the pristine tiles. The atmosphere seemed unusually tense in the room, though there was no patient currently on the operating table. There was nothing untoward to see, either. Chatting among themselves, the surgical nurses were collecting blood-stained swabs, flotsam and jetsam in kidney dishes and painstakingly cleaning the operating area. In a corner, the surgeon was scrubbing his forearms and hands.

Though he had his back turned to her and still wore a white surgical cap, Kitty recognised the dark clippered hair at the nape of his neck and the perfect V of James's natural hairline.

'Dr Williams!' She hadn't expected her old flame still to be on duty. Her heart skipped a beat.

James looked around, wearing a quizzical frown on his face. Under the bright lights, he looked uncharacteristically drawn. 'Nurse Longthorne. Whatever's the matter?'

As if happening upon him wasn't unexpected enough, a white-clad figure, crouching down close to the operating table, examining the anaesthetist's equipment, stood up suddenly and turned around at the sound of her name. It was her saviour from the snow. He beamed at her and blushed.

'Dr Collins!' Kitty said, looking from one man to the other.

Right at that moment, the friction between the two men was almost palpable. Or was she merely imagining things? Had Richard had the opportunity to speak to James about their impromptu coffee date? Or had James interrogated him about their arriving at the hospital together in his Hillman Minx? Of course not, she reasoned! Lives were at stake in the operating theatre. Both men had far better things to do than to exchange chit-chat about plain old Kitty Longthorne and her second-hand sheepskin boots. She felt guilty and silly for thinking such a thing under such grave circumstances.

'How lovely to see you again so soon, Kitty,' Richard said. 'Are you fully thawed?'

'I am. Yes. Thanks.' She felt her cheeks stinging hot with embarrassment. 'I didn't realise either of you would be here.'

'Ships passing in the night,' James said. 'I'm about to go off shift. The professor's delayed in the snow. Dr Collins, here, was just coming on, weren't you, old bean?' His words were friendly but his tone was cold.

'Well, I've got a patient on the trolley in the corridor,' she said breathlessly, pushing her own drama aside. 'Dora Mackie. A mother of five, found at the bottom of her stairs. Terrible head injury. But my immediate concern is a suspected collapsed lung. There's not a soul to be found in the emergency department. All the doctors are tending to snow-related calamities. So, forgive me for steaming down here without going through the necessary procedures, but –' She searched James's tired-looking but handsome face for understanding.

He nodded. 'Of course. I trust your judgement. Bring her straight in. Professor Baird-Murray isn't due for at least another twenty minutes. I'll see what I can do for her in the meantime.'

Kitty gestured to the ambulance men to wheel the unconscious patient into the theatre. They greeted James respectfully, almost bowing before him.

'Thank you, gentlemen,' he said. 'Do take care on the roads in this vile weather. You're doing a sterling job.'

The men nodded solemnly, leaving the theatre nursing staff to quickly prepare the operating table for the mortally ill Dora.

James lifted his new patient's eyelids, checking to see if her pupils reacted to the bright light that shone from the end of his small pen-torch. He performed small, simple tests of her reflexes to check for spinal injuries and seemed satisfied that there were none.

'Ideally, we need an X-ray to double check what's happening with that bang to the head,' he said. 'But this lung must be dealt with first.' He held his arm out towards the doors, indicating that it was time for Kitty to leave. 'Thank you, Nurse Longthorne. Your instincts were entirely correct. I hope to return Mrs Mackie to your good care on the ward soon.' He treated her to a flicker of a smile.

Kitty let the double doors to the operating theatre slap shut behind her. For a moment, she lingered by the window, looking in at the scene of brisk efficiency and total concentration as James gave his nursing staff instructions to prepare Dora's mottled chest for incision, and Richard held a mask over her face, sending her into a deep, deep sleep.

As her gaze moved from the anaesthetist to the surgeon, coming to rest on James, Kitty felt a sharp tap on her shoulder.

'And what do you think you're doing, ogling the men, Longthorne?'

Chapter 22

Kitty took a sharp intake of breath and spun around, expecting to see Sister Iris's sour face glaring at her. Instead, she giggled nervously.

'Vi! You're too good at impersonating people! You nearly gave me a heart attack!' she said to her flame-haired friend, who grinned mischievously. Kitty clasped her hand over her chest, covering the place where all her secret longing and emotional turmoil lurked. Had Violet really suspected that she'd been ogling James? 'I've just rushed an incoming patient straight to theatre. The emergency department's a nightmare with this deep freeze.'

Violet began to fidget with the buttons on her cape, barely glancing into the theatre at her fiancé. 'I think they should issue fur-lined capes, personally. We'll catch our deaths, going back to the nurses' home. And then where will they all be?'

They walked together down the corridor, Kitty leading the way, since she could already imagine the dressing down she would be given by Sister Iris for being late. 'How come you're not assisting in theatre? I haven't seen you in an age, because you're never on the wards.'

Smoothing her hair beneath her starched nurse's cap, the brilliance of Violet's pearly smile dimmed somewhat. 'It was James's idea, actually. I've been redeployed on the maternity ward. He said our being engaged and working together . . .'

She flicked the solitaire diamond ring on her wedding finger around so that momentarily, it looked like a wedding band. Then she stuffed her hand into her pocket – 'Was a conflict of interest.' The movement of cartilage within her thin neck betrayed a swallowing of pride. 'Now he's on the Board of Governors, he's no fun at all.' She closed her eyes briefly and laughed, though her laughter was hollow.

'How so?' Kitty asked.

'Everything changed when they passed that dratted NHS Act last year,' Violet said, trying and failing to sound breezy. 'He thinks because he's the youngest governor that he's got to be the perfect poster boy for the new health service. It's terribly boring. All he does is drone on about how intractable the likes of the professor are.'

'Well, he's not wrong there!' Kitty said. 'They're all desperate to cling onto their private practice.'

'Who can blame them? Daddy said the economy will be ruined if the nation's medical professionals become lowly paid lackeys of a Labour government overnight.'

'I'm not sure they'll be low-paid lack—'

'James thinks he's some kind of people's champion.' She tutted and rolled her eyes, then sniffed hard, as though mentally dismissing James's aspirations as nothing more than frivolous self-indulgence.

Kitty was just about to leap to James's defence, when Violet changed tack entirely.

'Oh, you'll never guess what! I've finally decided on a design for a wedding dress. Christian Dior has *just* launched his New Look.' Violet flapped her hand animatedly as she spoke. 'It's out of this world, Kitty. And Mummy wants me to go to a couturier in Paris that she knows. She's going to get me something made in white silk – à la Dior, of course.'

'Have you and James set a date, then?' Kitty asked, poised to part company with her friend at the bottom of the stairs. Silently, she counselled herself to keep calm and remember the unexpected date she'd just enjoyed with Richard Collins. There was life after James Williams. Or so it seemed.

Violet looked at the handrail. 'Err, not exactly, no. James says it's not appropriate, with him being so busy with his pioneering surgical techniques and being on the board and everything.' She smiled fleetingly, but it was all teeth and no mirth. 'His father is very keen that we tie the knot and get on with starting a family. My mother can't *wait* to announce the wedding arrangements in the *Tatler* and the *Telegraph*, but all in good time, I suppose. I'm twenty-six but at least I'm not an old spinster like you.' Her grin returned with all the brilliance of an operating-theatre light. She nudged Kitty in the upper arm and winked. 'Only joking, darling! Right, I'd better dash.'

As Kitty ascended the stairs to her ward, she batted aside the irritation at Violet's uncharitable comments – clearly designed to amuse her at Kitty's expense – to make sense of what had been said – or, rather, what hadn't been said. Despite her insinuations that they were on the brink of tying the knot, Violet still didn't have a date for the big day. Her wedding arrangements were currently all in her own wishful imagination. In fact, there was now a professional distance between Violet and James, at his instigation. That much was clear. Kitty wondered if she should take comfort in this news, given that Violet had stolen James from under her nose?

She shook her head and strode purposefully down to the ward.

'You're better than that, Kitty Longthorne,' she said beneath her breath. 'And look at poor Dora Mackie and what loving the wrong man has done for her. Maybe you'd do better by staying an old maid. Follow in Matron's impressive footsteps.'

Pushing the door to the ward open, Kitty's dreams of one day becoming Matron were immediately dashed by the thunderous look on Sister Iris's glowering face.

The formidable sister pointed to the ward clock. 'Wipe that smile off your face, Longthorne. What time do you call this, young lady?'

'The snow made me late. And I was tending to an emergency, sister. A woman needed to be rushed to theatre and I was the only staff member on hand. Ask Dr Williams! He's doing emergency surgery on her right now. I'm ever so sorry. It won't happen again.'

Several of the patients were craning their necks to see what the commotion was all about. Kitty smiled weakly at them, wishing she could will the heat from her cheeks. It didn't do to show Sister Iris any kind of weakness.

'The new junior is in the sluice room. We've got gastro-enteritis in a side room. You'd better get going before I report you to Matron.'

Sister Iris turned on her heel and headed off down the ward. Kitty started to make her way to the sluice room when she heard Iris's barking voice.

'Schwartz, you stupid, stupid girl! Can't you read, you Dummkopf Kraut? This man is nil by mouth!'

Kitty turned round to witness the toe-curling spectacle of Sister Iris, bearing down on the tiny Lily within earshot of the entire ward. Lily visibly shrank from the blast of her superior's temper tantrum.

'I wasn't giving him a drink, sister,' Lily said in English that was flawless but for her accent. 'I was only moistening his lips. The patient was so uncomfortable. I didn't think it would do any harm.' Lily was wringing her hands, her head hanging dejectedly.

'Idiot! What is the point of having protocols if you're going to ignore them?'

Kitty was torn. She knew she shouldn't confront a senior member of nursing staff, undermining her authority by sticking up for her friend. Tears started to splash onto the highly polished parquet around Lily's feet, however.

'Come on, now, Kitty. Don't get involved,' Kitty whispered to herself. She chewed on her lip and tried to bite her tongue, but it was no good. She knew what she was witnessing was terribly unjust. *Don't get involved?* The mocking voice of her conscience resounded inside her head. *What are you? A doormat? Stand up and be counted for once in your life!*

Angry at Sister Iris, and at Violet, and at all of those women who thought they could belittle and mock others just to make themselves feel better about their own lives, and angry at all of those men like her father, who thought they could shout or beat their womenfolk into submission, Kitty marched down the ward towards the commotion. Sister Iris was still bellowing her dissatisfaction at Lily. Lily stood like a rag doll that had had its stuffing pulled out by a spoiled child, her shoulders quaking with sorrow.

'Is there a problem, here?' Kitty asked, locking eyes with Sister Iris and slipping her hand onto Lily's shoulder.

Sister Iris was momentarily non-plussed. She looked at Kitty, appearing confused with a fading sneer on her lips. 'I beg your pardon.'

Kitty stood as straight as she could, though she was still a good few inches shorter than Iris. 'Only, you seem rather cross at Nurse Schwartz for doing exactly what Matron trained us to do – to care for the patient as well as we can and to use our initiative.'

The promontory of Sister Iris's brow seemed to bulge like a brewing storm cloud. 'How *dare* you challenge my authority?' she said, dropping the volume of her voice to deadly quiet.

'Oh, I dare,' Kitty said. 'Nurse Schwartz doesn't deserve your dressing down. She was dutifully tending to her patient's needs, weren't you, Lily?'

Lily nodded. 'I was only doing my best.'

'And she's not a Dummkopf Kraut. She's an intelligent, qualified nurse.'

'If she's not a Kraut, then what is she?' Sister Iris said. 'Scotch mist?'

'The war's over, Sister Iris. There's no need to be nasty about Lily's origins. Her parents came to this country as refugees, not Nazis. Don't you think that standing here at the foot of a sick patient's bed, bellowing at a junior member of staff while she's crying her eyes out might give the hospital a bad name? People come here to get medical care. What you're doing looks pretty uncaring to me.' Where had the words come from? Kitty had no idea. She'd just opened her mouth and out they'd trotted. She knew she should be frightened of Sister Iris's inevitable wrath, but she wasn't. At that moment, Kitty's stomach felt like it was buzzing with the energy of a thousand bees, defending their hive. The cold, her hunger and fatigue were all forgotten.

Without waiting for a response, Kitty took Lily by the hand and marched back towards the sluice room. 'Come on, Lil. Take a breather. Get yourself cleaned up. I'll shoulder anything coming my way. The way I feel right now, I could happily ram Sister Iris's cap right—'

Just as Kitty was about to reveal her intentions to Lily, she felt a strong hand grip her shoulder.

'Not so fast, young lady,' Sister Iris said. 'Did you really think I was going to take that kind of cheek lying down? Off *you*, of all people?'

'Get off me,' Kitty said, trying to wriggle free. 'I haven't done anything wrong.'

Her protestations were to no avail. Kitty and Lily were both frog-marched to Matron, who was deep in conversation with Professor Baird-Murray in the staffroom.

'I say! What's all this, then?' Professor Baird-Murray said, straightening his slacks as he adjusted his position in his chair.

Matron peered round at them, her gaze coming to rest on Kitty. She narrowed her eyes and raised an eyebrow.

'Insubordination!' Sister Iris shouted by means of an explanation. 'You wouldn't believe the tirade of verbal abuse I've just endured from Longthorne, here.'

Professor Baird-Murray teased a beautiful gold pocket watch from the breast pocket of his herringbone tweed jacket, registered the time with a disbelieving snort, and rose from his armchair. 'I'm afraid I can't be party to such frivolity,' he said in his rasping smoker's voice. 'Surgery awaits! I'll leave these high-spirited gals in your capable hands, matron.'

As he left the staffroom, a lingering smell of tobacco, mothballs and TCP remained.

'Sister Iris,' Matron said, smoothing her skirt over her substantial knees. 'Was it really necessary to interrupt an important discussion about the running of the hospital, in this time of dire need, with mundane staffing issues?'

Sister Iris opened her mouth to respond, but Matron raised her hand for silence.

'Has either nurse harmed a patient or endangered a life?'

'Schwartz moistened the lips of . . .' The words died on Iris's tongue. 'No.'

Matron got to her feet with a grunt. 'We're woefully understaffed and overstretched, Sister Iris. I'll leave it to you to punish any unseemly behaviour of the nurses under your jurisdiction as you see fit, but really, aren't we all too busy to be taking time out of our shifts for things that can be dealt with on the ward?' She angled her head towards Sister Iris like a stern school ma'am, waiting for a reaction from a wayward child who had just been told off for bickering in the playground.

When they returned to the ward in silence, it was clear that Sister Iris was fuming.

As they approached the doors, she said, 'You can both add a couple of hours onto your shifts for the rest of the week.'

Kitty knew better than to keep the argument going. 'Yes, sister. Absolutely.' She nudged Lily.

'Of course, sister.' Lily glanced at Kitty, mouthing a silent *thank you* once Iris's back was turned.

Grabbing her friend's hand and squeezing it in solidarity, Kitty felt good to have stood up to a woman who had been abusing her power for all the years that she had worked at Park Hospital. If she could face down Sister Iris, perhaps she could also confront her father.

Chapter 23

An hour or so later, as Kitty emerged from a gruesome session of sluicing bedpans and soiled bedding, the doors to the ward swung open to reveal a patient on a trolley, being pushed by two orderlies and accompanied by a theatre nurse. Making a beeline for Sister Iris, who was seated at her desk in her makeshift office with the door open, the theatre nurse carried a sheaf of notes with her. She handed them to Iris and they had a brief exchange, just out of Kitty's earshot.

'Oh, here we go,' Lily said, mopping her way closer to Kitty to get a good look at the incoming admission. 'First new one in a few days. I wonder who we're getting.'

Catching a glimpse of the bandaged head and livid purple bruising to her face, Kitty hazarded a guess. 'I think it's Dora Mackie. The woman I rushed into theatre with a suspected broken rib and collapsed lung. If she's just come up from surgery, she must be out of the woods. I hope so.'

As the trolley trundled past, Kitty saw that it was indeed Dora Mackie beneath the oxygen mask. Despite the bruising, her skin was a better colour. She was wheeled over to the vacant bed that she and Lily had recently remade with precision.

'Longthorne! Schwartz! Attend to the new patient!' Sister Iris shouted through the office door, not even bothering to rise from her desk chair. 'She'll need supervision throughout the night.'

Ignoring the sour expression on Iris's face as they made their way past the Sister's office, Kitty and Lily approached Dora. She was sleeping, now.

'Let's get her in bed. See how she goes through the night,' Kitty said. 'I'm happy to watch her. With a head wound like that, it's anyone's guess how she'll be when she wakes.'

Assisted by Lily, Kitty pushed the trolley closer to the bed. They slid panels beneath the patient and deftly transferred her from the trolley to the bed with minimum fuss, though Kitty winced when the poor woman yelped in pain in her sleep.

Once she'd hooked her breathing apparatus up to a new cylinder of oxygen, she arranged the bag of fluid on the drip stand at the head of the bed and checked that the tubing and needle hadn't been disturbed during the transfer process. Kitty retrieved Dora's notes and read through them. Her suspicions had been correct. Dora had indeed received several blows to the head, the worst of which seemed to have come from a tumble down the stairs. With no bleed on the brain, she'd been lucky enough to escape with a bad concussion. Her rib *had* been cracked and had punctured the lung. What was inconclusive, however, was how Dora had sustained her injuries. Kitty knew that there was no way that a tumble down the stairs was the only mishap that had befallen her patient.

At three in the morning, Dora finally woke. Kitty was standing by her bedside as her lashes started to flutter.

'Hello,' Kitty said, fastening a clean white starched apron behind her back. 'You won't remember me. I'm the nurse who took care of you when you first arrived in the ambulance.'

Dora looked at her with unfocussed eyes and smiled weakly. She tried to pull off her oxygen mask to speak, but seemingly lacked the energy to do more than poke at it with a bloodied fingernail. 'They said I was rushed in by an angel. So you're her?' Her voice was muffled by the hiss of oxygen entering the mask that covered her nose and mouth. She spoke slowly and ponderously, as though the words were hard to nail down – clearly still very concussed.

Kitty chuckled. 'Well, I am the nurse who brought you in, but I'm not sure about being an angel.'

'Take no notice,' Lily said to Dora as she drew close to greet Kitty's new charge. 'She definitely is an angel, this one!'

Kitty rolled her eyes at Lily, then turned to her patient. She started to adjust her pillows. 'Come on, Mrs Mackie. Let's get you more comfortable.'

'Call me Dora, love.'

'Tell me, do you have any family to visit you, Dora?' Kitty asked.

Dora looked blankly at the foot of the bed. Her eyes widened as though something important had only just occurred to her. 'My babies! I've got five of 'em. Such beauties. I hope he's looking after them, my old man. I hope to Christ he's keeping them fed and warm.' Her bruised face suddenly crumpled into an expression of pure woe and worry. 'Oh, is there any way someone can check on my babies? Please, nurse!' She grabbed at Kitty's apron, pulling her close. She dropped her woozy-sounding voice to a whisper. 'I need to know they're safe, only my Francis isn't very . . . He gets wound up by the noise and the mess, you know? I mean, can you imagine what a trial it is for a grown man to live under the same roof as all those little'uns?'

'Don't you have a mother or a sister who's looking after them while you're in here?' Kitty asked. She exchanged a knowing glance with Lily, who stood at the foot of the next bed, clearly eavesdropping and pretending to read a sleeping patient's notes.

Dora sounded beset by panic. 'My poor mam . . .'

'What about your mam?'

'She – she died in the Blitz. My auntie's miles away in Rawtenstall. No. There's nobody but my neighbour, Mrs –' She frowned and winced. 'I can't remember her name. It's on the tip of my tongue.'

Calculating how long it would take five small children to die from hypothermia, starvation, dehydration or some other dreadful misadventure that might arise as a result of neglect or just the biting, never-ending cold, Kitty realised she had yet another emergency on her hands. Should she get involved personally and drop in at Dora's home? Was it possible that Sister Iris would let her off her shift at the normal time, rather than insist she complete the daily extra two hours that had been added on as a disciplinary measure?

She glanced over at Sister Iris, who was seated at the bedside of a sleeping old woman, engrossed in reading a novel, barely concealed behind the patients' notes. No, expecting empathy or leniency from that battle-axe was a fool's errand, and this was the sort of case where other hospital staff could bring their professional expertise to bear.

'I can have a word with the health visitor,' Kitty offered. 'Perhaps she'll drop by to check on your family.'

'No! No health visitors.' There was alarm in Dora's voice.

'But your youngest children must be under two. Surely, they're still being monitored by—'

'My babies don't need no monitoring. They're well-fed and kept clean. They want for nowt.'

But Dora herself seemed excessively thin and had arrived at the hospital in the ambulance, dressed in dirty and ill-fitting clothes that suggested jumble-sale cast-offs and poor access to washing facilities. If the mother was undernourished and neglected, how likely was it that the children were, too? 'How about I speak to one of the ladies from the Institute of Almoners? They do some valuable social work with—'

'My Francis doesn't like strangers digging their beaks into our business. He's a very private man. A war hero like him doesn't need no charity.'

Her slurred, concussed speech notwithstanding, Dora's reluctance to have authorities poking around was clear – small wonder, if *my Francis* was a tyrant in the home and if their housing was inadequate for quite so many young children.

'Listen. I've got your address on file,' Kitty said, patting Dora's hand gently. 'I'll nip round in the morning when my shift's finished. I'll check on them all personally. How's that?'

Dora nodded and squeezed Kitty's hand. 'Bless you. I'd never forgive myself if anything happened to my kiddies. Not that it would.'

Checking her nurse's watch, Kitty smiled. Another seven hours of her extended shift remained. 'Visiting time's tomorrow. Who knows? Maybe Mr Mackie will bring the children to see you.'

Dora inhaled sharply. 'I don't want them chancing it in this snow. It's dangerous out there. They'll slip or freeze to death.'

Was she genuinely concerned for their safety, or was she also terrified at the prospect of Mr Mackie turning up at the hospital? Though taking an interest in patients' private lives was not within her jurisdiction, given Dora's clear refusal to have health visitors or the almoners involved, Kitty felt compelled to find out more.

'Don't you fret, Dora,' Kitty said, patting the woman's shaking hand. 'I'll bob round in the morning and check on them.'

'Tell them not to come!'

'I'll tell them. Now, you get some rest. You've a nasty concussion and your oxygen levels still aren't marvellous.'

After a short while, Kitty saw Dora's battered body start to relax. Her head lolled to the left and her eyes finally closed. She was asleep.

As Kitty became almost entranced by the hiss and whine of Dora's breathing apparatus, thinking about her own impossible, impassable family situation, an uneventful hour passed. The silence on the ward was punctured only by the elderly woman diagonally opposite, who'd wandered off in the snow, thanks to her advanced dementia, and who now moaned intermittently in her troubled half-sleep, still believing she was in the midst of the Blitz. Kitty enjoyed the night shifts, precisely because they were generally a gentler time of the day, with the lights on low and the patients snoring.

When a quarter to six came round, however, Kitty was shaken out of a trance-like stupor by the sound of laboured gurgling. She looked over at her charge and saw that Dora had turned an alarming blue-grey colour.

Kitty rushed over to Sister Iris, speaking quietly but quickly into her ear. 'Dora Mackie is in trouble,' she said. 'I think her lung has collapsed again.'

Sister Iris nodded briskly and hastened with Kitty back to Dora's bedside. As she examined Dora, checking that her oxygen was still coming through and feeling for her pulse, Kitty's heartbeat galloped along at a frenzied pace.

'This woman isn't going to survive,' Sister Iris said. 'Get Mr Galbraith, girl! Hurry!'

Mr Galbraith was a new arrival to the Park Hospital staff from King's Hospital, London. He was a specialist in cardiothoracic medicine famed for successfully removing the cancerous portion of a lung in a patient, with no need for further therapy or treatment beyond bedrest and abstinence from tobacco. Kitty had overheard Professor Baird-Murray singing his praises in the staffroom. Surely, this scalpel-wielding genius was the man who could save Dora Mackie.

As Kitty ran through the freezing cold corridors, she prayed under her breath. 'Please let me save her. Please, God. Please don't let Mam die,' she whispered to the distempered brick walls.

It was then that she realised that somehow her own mother had become linked to Dora, in her anguished, overburdened mind. Was it the brow-beating husband? The grinding poverty? The woman having to fend for her children like a lioness defending her cubs against terrible odds?

'Not on my shift, Dora. You're not dying tonight, love.'

Kitty happened upon the lung surgeon in his office. He was a thin, sharply dressed man with a shining bald pate and a pencil moustache, surrounded by administrative clutter and watched over by a full-length skeleton that hung in the corner. She explained the situation.

Gathering some instruments into his doctor's bag, Mr Galbraith followed her back up to the ward.

When they arrived, the other patients were beginning to stir. Kitty drew aside the curtain to Dora's cubicle to find her lying perfectly still on her bed. Her mask had been removed; her skin was a grim colour.

Mr Galbraith felt for her pulse and pursed his lips. 'Draw the curtain, Nurse Kitty. Be quick. Death is standing over this bed and I have no time for the ugly old devil.'

Chapter 24

'I think I've done all I can for her,' Galbraith said, carefully tying off the stitches that closed the incision he'd made in her chest.

Kitty looked down at Dora, whose colour had returned somewhat and whose chest rose and fell once more, though she was unconscious. 'You saved her.'

'We'll see.' Galbraith removed his blood-splattered white coat and made for the sink. He methodically started to wash his hands. The water ran scarlet down the plughole. 'This woman had a raging respiratory infection that had started up long before she was admitted to casualty. She's in dire health. It's a small wonder that there have been complications. But I'm leaving her under your excellent care. Make sure she gets her antibiotics, nurse, and we'll see how fate treats her.'

Satisfied that Dora's condition was now stable, Kitty began to clean up after the impromptu surgery. Collecting the bucket from the sluice room, she ran boiling hot water into it and threw in a good measure of disinfectant. She was just soaking the mop in the bucket and gathering together some clean rags when Sister Iris appeared in the doorway.

'What a commotion,' the sister said, blinking fast through those ugly glasses she wore. 'I don't like commotion on my shift.'

Feeling exhaustion and frayed nerves gnawing away at her composure, Kitty tried and failed to bite her tongue. 'We're here to save lives, aren't we? Maybe I'd also rather sit reading a book on the sly than assist in emergency surgery, but *I* trained to look after the sick and wounded. It's my job, and I'll be damned if I don't do it properly.'

She noisily hefted the clanking bucket past Sister Iris, who stood open mouthed for the briefest of moments.

'How dare you speak to me like that, young lady,' the sister said, hands on her hips. 'I don't know what you're insinuating! This kind of insubordination is—'

'Oh, this old chestnut, *again*? I don't have time for it, Iris,' Kitty said. 'I've got cleaning to do, and then I've got to finish all my other shift duties. So, if you're going to run with tales to Matron a second time, I suggest you just get on and do it.'

Kitty heard the sharp intake of breath from her superior, but didn't wait around to see the undoubted look of outrage and disgust on her doughy face.

I don't care what happens, Kitty thought. *I'm in the right. And if Matron was going to sack me, she'd have done it by now. I've got to stand up and be counted, because if I'm ever to be promoted, I need the likes of Iris to treat me with respect.* Despite the morale-boosting pep-talk she was mentally giving herself, Kitty's hands shook as she began her clean-up around Dora's bed.

Count to twenty, she counselled herself, as Dora's life-saving apparatus hissed and whined in time with her own laboured heartbeat. *One, two, three . . .*

Realising that Iris had retreated back into her office and had closed the door, Kitty locked eyes with Lily, who was feeding breakfast to a patient across the way, and couldn't quite stifle a nervous giggle.

'You're my heroine!' Lily whispered, mischievous delight apparent in her broad grin. 'Marlene Dietrich has got nothing on you!'

Finishing up her cleaning task, Kitty said, 'You think that was daring. Watch this!'

The clock on the wall said her shift had ended some twenty minutes earlier. Dora was sleeping, and the dayshift nurses were already beginning their morning duties at the top of the ward. Kitty marched to Sister Iris's office and knocked smartly on the door. Sister Iris was sitting at her makeshift desk, eating a bacon sandwich.

'I'm going now,' Kitty said.

'You've got another two hours,' Iris said, the half-chewed food visible as she spoke with her mouth full.

'I'm not doing it. I'm sorry. I have personal commitments, and this shift has left me wiped out. Lily's watching Dora Mackie, until the dayshift nurse makes her way down the ward. I'm off. See you tonight.'

Sister Iris stood abruptly, scraping her chair along the floor noisily. 'I –' She looked down at her sandwich and set it back on her side plate. Then she laced her hands together over her belly. 'I'm –' Was she going to apologise? 'See you this evening, Longthorne. Enjoy your well-earned rest.'

Finally, the bully had backed down. Suddenly, Kitty could no longer feel the icy chill of the morning air, permeating the ward. She was flushed warm with moral triumph and marched along the corridors of the hospital, towards the main entrance, with a spring in her aching feet.

Fiddling with the buttons on her nurse's cape and recalling in delicious detail the look of defeat on the dreaded Iris's face, Kitty was so locked in a world of her own that she didn't see the smartly dressed man, standing at the bottom of the stairs until she walked into him.

'I say, Kitty! Steady on!' It was James. He took her hand as though he were stopping her from falling, though she was perfectly grounded. For a change, he wasn't wearing his white coat but a smartly tailored grey gabardine suit.

Kitty pulled her hand away, feeling her cheeks glow. 'Sorry! Sorry. I was miles away.' She blinked hard and bit her lip, talking too quickly. 'Long shift. And I've got to get to Stretford to go and check on Dora Mackie's children. It could take hours in this dratted weather.'

The glow coming through the window from the snowy blanket that smothered everything outside gave James an unhealthy pallor and made the distempered walls almost too dazzling so that she had to squint.

'Why on earth are you making home visits to check on patients' children? Can't the health visitor or the almoners get involved?'

Kitty shook her head. 'The woman's petrified of authorities. You know the story, surely! The husband comes home from war and can't settle.'

James nodded sagely. 'No more routine, no purpose. It's a shock to the system to be a family man again after years of the camaraderie of only men.'

'Problem is, there's nowhere for that battlefield aggression to go anymore, so the children and womenfolk are the ones who get it in the neck.'

'The hidden price of valour. I can give men like your brother new faces but I can't fix what's in here' – he pointed to his head – 'or here.' He pointed to his heart. He stuffed his hands into his pockets awkwardly. 'Look, I would offer to come with you, but I've a board meeting.' He checked his gold wristwatch and sighed. His eyes met hers. 'Do be careful, Kitty. If Mrs Mackie's husband is a thug . . .'

Kitty stood a little taller and straighter, focussing on the neat parting in James's black hair. 'I'm not Violet, as we both know. I don't need chaperoning or misplaced chivalry. I hope your meeting goes well.'

With that, she continued resolutely on her way back to the nurses' home, wondering if the exhaustion of doing nightshifts and the terrible biting cold of the weather had finally got to her. The last thing she wanted to do was make an enemy of the man she'd loved – still loved. But Kitty felt as though the trials of her post-war life were turning her into somebody stronger and more daring.

Catching sight of her new admirer, Richard Collins, crossing from one side of the hospital to the other, Kitty ducked out of view and giggled to herself. She felt like a spy. She felt like a rebel. It was intoxicating.

Chapter 25

'Hello! Is there anyone home?' Kitty asked, banging on the front door for a third time. A large curl of flaking red paint dislodged itself and drifted down onto the virgin snow on the doorstep.

No footprints. Perhaps nobody had entered or left the house since Dora had been taken away in the ambulance, Kitty calculated. She pushed open the letterbox, trying to glimpse what lay beyond. As with all of the Victorian terraces in the area, the front door immediately opened onto a square living room. What she could see was a dank, dark and cluttered mess with dirty clothing and children's paraphernalia strewn everywhere her eye rested.

'Mr Mackie! Are you there?'

There was no answer, though Kitty looked up, feeling that she was being watched from the window above, thick with hoarfrost and grime. She shivered uncontrollably in her too-thin coat and her second-hand sheepskin boots, which were starting to let moisture in.

Presently the neighbouring front door opened and a jolly-faced fat woman peered out.

'You looking for Dora?' she asked in a gruff voice that belied her friendly appearance.

Kitty shook her head. 'Mr Mackie. I wanted to check on the children.'

The neighbour's apparent joviality slid from her face. She looked downright hostile. 'You some health visitor? Some do-gooder sticking their beak in? We don't like that sort around here, telling us how we should be living and then doing nowt to help.'

'No.' Kitty held her gloved hands up, feeling suddenly dizzy with fatigue. 'Nothing like that. I'm the nurse that's been looking after Dora in hospital. She came in last night after a fall down the stairs. She asked me to come and check on the children.'

The neighbour looked down her ruddy nose at Kitty, as if assessing her. She nodded abruptly and opened her door wide. 'The kiddies are with me. You'd better come in. They're a right handful and I could do with an adult to speak to for five minutes over a brew. I feel like I'm losing my marbles.'

Kitty looked up and down the snow-bound street, still feeling like she was being observed. She stepped over the threshold and through a glazed door into the neighbour's front room. Immediately, she was assailed by the sound of screaming small children and the smell of soiled nappies. The place was freezing cold but spotless. There, in the middle of the living room, was a blue wooden playpen containing all of Dora's children, with the baby lying on a crocheted blanket in the middle, oblivious to his tiny siblings who clung to the bars, tearful and streaming with snot.

'Mine are all grown-up,' the neighbour said. 'My son fought in the war.' Her ruddy cheeks paled. 'Dunkirk landings.' She breathed in deeply through her nose.

On the mantelpiece above a barely smouldering fire, Kitty noticed a framed portrait of an elegant-looking young man in uniform, gazing into the middle distance. He had his mother's twinkling eyes. The ornate Victorian frame – conceivably an heirloom but perhaps equally likely a jumble-sale find or bomb-site salvage – had been painted black. It was the grandest thing in the room that was otherwise furnished with mismatched floral threadbare chairs and a sofa, the large 1930s wooden wireless taking pride of place in the recess by the fireplace atop an old wooden crate, partly covered with an embroidered cloth. The floor was wooden planks; scrubbed clean and covered with a rag rug. Kitty could feel the icy wind whipping up through the cracks between the floorboards from the cellar. The place smelled of bleach, barely covering the sharp tang of damp.

'I'm sorry for your loss,' she said. 'My brother was in a prisoner-of-war camp in Japan. Blown up on the boat home and left with shocking disfigurements. Sometimes I think it would have been better if he'd never returned.'

Their shared moment of grief was interrupted by the barking cough of the middle child – a girl of about three with golden-blonde curls and the florid complexion of a toddler running a fever. She coughed and coughed and vomited over her knitted cardigan.

'Oh, here she goes again!' the neighbour said. 'Come on, Polly. Let's get you cleaned up, little lamb.' She scooped up the child and whisked her off to the kitchen.

Though she was reluctant to leave the other children behind, Kitty reasoned they were at least safe, so she followed her hostess through to the back. The kitchen had the appearance of a makeshift sluice room. The sturdy pine table that took up half of the room was covered in clean nappy-changing paraphernalia: cotton wool, talcum powder, a bottle of Johnson's baby lotion and a big tub of zinc and castor oil. On the stove, a large pot was boiling away. The roiling steam from it smelled strongly of Milton washing fluid, fogging up the tall kitchen window which showed little of the white-out in the backyard beyond. No doubt the steel cooking pot contained a strange stew of terry towelling nappies, such as the ones in the pile laid out on the table. Above the table hung a wooden drying rack, loaded with pristine children's clothes. There was an additional clothes horse, loaded with white terry towelling squares that had been wedged in the corner by the back door, hemmed in by a giant old pram full of folded laundry.

'It's a bugger looking after all these babies,' the neighbour said, deftly stripping the wriggling small girl of her soiled clothing with one hand. In the other, she held a battered-looking cuddly toy of sorts, fashioned from a ball of old socks, with black glass buttons for eyes and mouth, nose and whiskers dog-stitched on in wool. She waved it above the child's head in a desperate bid to jolly her out of her tantrum. 'I've done my whack, see –' she inclined her head towards the giant pram – 'and I can't get to the wash house, so my scullery's turned into the Hanging Gardens of Babylon. Nowt dries in this flaming weather. It's a nightmare. And this is just one day!'

'Here, let me help,' Kitty said, taking the toy and allowing the little girl to clutch it in her freshly wiped hands. Her inflamed cheeks were burning hot. The snot encrusted around her nose was green. Kitty took a soft cloth and dipped it into the bowl of warm water. She wiped the little girl's face clean, noticing, as she brushed her blonde curls aside, that the child's hair was peppered with small brown dots. 'This little girl is very ill. And she's got nits!'

'Ha! You're telling me,' the neighbour said, tweezering a juicy head louse from the girl's scalp between her fingernails and popping it. 'They're all crawling with 'em.' She pointed to her own tightly plaited hair, pinned closely to her head and covered with a sheer, turbaned scarf. 'Why do you think I've got my hair like this? The last thing I need at my age is nits. I've still got a comb from when mine were little, but what I need is some Derbac soap. Give these little'uns a proper tubbing. Can I get to the shops, though, with screaming tots to look after? Can I, heckers like! It's a miracle Dora keeps them alive. She's been popping them out since they moved here, when she was big with her eldest. One every nine or ten months. A pair of twins, and then the baby. They're like rabbits, him and her. It's scandalous, if you ask me.'

'Does Mr Mackie not help?'

The neighbour gave a sour-sounding laugh. She raised an eyebrow and opened her mouth to speak. Then she seemed to think better of it and pressed her thin lips together briefly. 'Let's just say, Mr Mackie's handy, but not with his own children.'

'Handy with his fists?'

Again, the neighbour's lips parted and then snapped shut like a defensive clam. 'Loose lips sink ships,' she said finally. 'I'm not going to be responsible for bringing the authorities to Dora's door, and her maybe having her children taken away.'

Kitty placed a placatory hand on the neighbour's meaty arm as she hefted the clean toddler into her arms and onto her hip. 'Please. If you think Dora's life is in danger, you have to tell someone. Who's going to look after her family if she's murdered?'

The neighbour frowned and studied Kitty's face momentarily. 'I'm no grass. You posh people might do that kind of thing, but, around here, we watch each other's backs.'

Feeling the heat of irritation starting to rise within her like mercury in a thermometer, Kitty narrowed her eyes. 'My family's from Hulme, love. Stretford's hoi polloi compared to where I lived before a doodlebug flattened our street. Just because I'm a nurse, don't think I don't know what it is to rough it. My mam and dad lived in one of the only houses left standing in a Chorlton-on-Medlock bomb site after VE day. No running water. No electricity. I've seen grander tents. Now, they're living near Strangeways, and my mam's sewing raincoats by day and pressing cap-linings in a sweatshop by night.'

The woman curled her lip in disgust. 'It's rank around there.'

'I've got news for you. The whole country's on its knees, and the ones who are suffering worst are women like Dora and their children. They're ill and they can't afford the doctor. They can't afford to eat. They can't afford to heat their homes.' Kitty thought briefly of her new admirer with his Hillman Minx that had almost certainly cost the same as a house. A small wave of disgust lapped close to her freezing feet, stuffed in her second-hand boots.

The neighbour set the clean and placated little girl back in the playpen and plucked out the next child down – one of the twins. She cradled his head against her ample bosom. 'We're all sleeping with coats on the bed and burning whatever we can get our hands on,' she said ruefully. 'I put my dead son's wardrobe on the fire two days ago. Now, give us a hand with these babies, make us a brew or take yourself back to Park Hospital. Your choice.'

'Of course,' Kitty said, realising that even her working-class credentials would not grant her a free pass into this tight-knit community.

Swallowing her fatigue and frustration down, she spent the next hour of her free time helping Dora's neighbour tend to the children. They enjoyed a cup of tea in jam jars, exchanging tales of surviving the Blitz and the rigors of rationing, before Kitty bid her new acquaintance farewell.

As she stood on the snowy doorstep, squinting in the blinding white light as fresh, fat flakes fluttered down, she turned to the woman. 'So, Mr Mackie's not shown his face since the accident? At least tell me that much.'

The woman had been just about to close her front door, but she paused, leaving a six-inch crack. 'He'll be gambling,' she said. 'Or sleeping it off somewhere. He knows I'll have taken his kids. I always do. I'm right soft like that. We won't be seeing him around here 'til Dora's back and fit to make his tea.'

Kitty nodded and smiled. *I always do.* So, this wasn't a one-off. 'Thanks. You're a kind soul.' She put her collar up against the biting cold and left.

Chapter 26

Wending her way up the slippery road towards the bus stop, Kitty started to formulate a plan – a way in which she might be of practical help to Dora, without putting her safety in jeopardy by reporting her situation to the authorities. She imagined that a thug like Mackie would beat his wife even harder if he thought she was running with tales. Men were proud. They were used to being right. Men liked their authority in their own home to go unchallenged – especially by women. Wasn't Kitty's own father cut from similar cloth? No, if Kitty were to help, she'd have to be cunning and dress intervention up as reward.

Returning to the hospital took two hours in the terrible downpour of snow, but though she was desperate for sleep and had nodded off several times on the bus, Kitty dragged her freezing, leaden body back into the relative warmth of the hospital. She found who she was looking for in the staffroom. He was sitting with several other doctors, shrouded in a choking yellow fug of their cigar and pipe smoke and engaged in what appeared to be a heated debate.

'Gentlemen!' one of the senior consultants said. 'We should absolutely dig our heels in at Park Hospital. Young Dr Williams here is showing all the zeal and lack of consideration of a Bolshevik. How am I to put my boy through Oxford if I'm just another functionary on a fixed salary? No private practice? Just a worker on the payroll of a Labour government, dependent on some wonk in Westminster for a handout? If I'd wanted to spend my life on my knees, I'd have joined the Civil Service, eh? What?'

There was a round of applause from some of the other senior consultants and raucous cheering, as though they were at some boyish debate club at a boarding school. Kitty tried to attract James's attention but he was staring blankly ahead, the sinews in his jaw flinching and his knuckles whitening as he gripped his knees.

'I say,' he said, 'I'll not have you call me a Bolshevik, Basil, just because I have a mandate to push forward plans—'

'This fool is sinking the ship! Throw him overboard!' one of the other doctors said, puffing away at his pipe as he applied a lit match to the tobacco. He threw the spent match dramatically into a full ashtray.

'The National Health Service is coming to Park Hospital, Charles, whether you like it or not. Manchester is gasping its last, thanks to poor housing and failing—'

'Change for change's sake!' Basil shouted above James. 'Bally load of idiots in Whitehall think they know better than us. Ha!'

Kitty had to interrupt. She cleared her throat and caught James's eye. 'Dr Williams, can I have a word with you about a patient, please?'

James smiled brightly and leaped from his chair. 'Do excuse me, gentlemen. I'll leave you to your pointless procrastination and pipe smoking. Toodle pip!'

Unexpectedly, he grabbed her by the elbow and whisked her out of the stuffy staffroom, into the corridor. Kitty blushed.

'Oh, James!' Reluctantly, she shook him loose, noticing that he looked rather crestfallen.

'My apologies. That was very forward of me.'

She relished his touch, but it wouldn't do to let the heart-breaker know her feelings could be toyed with. 'I don't think Violet would like to see you flinging me around as though we were jitterbugging.'

'No.' He chewed the inside of his cheek and his eyebrows knitted together. 'Quite.' Then his expression brightened. 'But I was cornered in there, and after a morning of board meetings – I'd rather have been in surgery – I couldn't bear any more heated debate with the dinosaurs.' He laced his hands together in front of him. A rebellious smile twitched at the corners of his mouth. He bowed slightly. 'So, thank you for saving me, Nurse Kitty.'

Was he flirting or just being friendly? She couldn't tell. Damn James Williams and his mixed messages! 'I was looking for you, actually,' she said, feeling like a lumpy old washerwoman in her heavy winter coat. Would James notice that she was wearing Violet's hand-me-down boots, tied with string? If he had, he didn't show it.

'Sounds intriguing. Do tell me more.'

Together, they walked slowly along the draughty corridor, the soles of their shoes squeaking on the spotless floor.

'About Dora Mackie . . .'

James nodded. 'Go on.'

'Well, I've just come back from visiting her house.'

'Her husband wasn't there, was he? Oh, Kitty. I really wish you wouldn't get involved in patients' personal lives. All we can do is treat them to the best of our ability and send them on their way. The rest is the jurisdiction of—'

'Her children are sick, James. They've got respiratory illnesses. They're malnourished. When they weren't screaming, they were withdrawn and skittish.'

'If women like Dora opt to stay with bad men—'

Coming to a halt, Kitty rounded on James. She glared at him, willing the angry words to arrange themselves in an articulate manner. 'Do you really think working-class women have an option to leave, when they're lumbered with husbands who beat them into submission? Where's a woman like Dora going to get enough money to support her family? She's a step away from the poorhouse.'

'Times are changing, Kitty. We're at the dawn of the Welfare State.' He sounded jubilant and important. 'Poorhouse, indeed! This isn't 1910!'

'All right, then. She's a step away from destitution, whichever way you look at it. And her and her children are suffering. Judging by the way they were coughing, if they've not got TB, they'll be lucky. Maybe they'll get away with a chest infection that could be treated, or asthma . . . – *if* they can scrape together enough money for the doctor. They live in the direst of circumstances, James.'

'We're medical people, Kitty. Not landlords. And not wealthy philanthropists who can wave a magic wand. Much as I wish we could, we can't rehouse them. That's beyond our scope. Speak to the almoners.'

'But surely we can do *something* for them. Get them away from the squalor and that beast, Mr Mackie, just for a few weeks? Take them on a holiday to the mountains!'

'Mountains? Like the Highlands or the Lake District – in the middle of the coldest winter for eons? How fanciful and romantic you are, Kitty Longthorne.'

'I'm not romanticising, James. I'm being practical. People within spitting distance of the hospital are dying for the want of fresh air. Women and children. I don't know about you, but I chose this job to save lives. *You're* in a position of power and influence, Dr Dawn-of-a-New-Era! What are you going to do about it?'

Chapter 27

'Longthorne!' There was an insistent knock at the door to Kitty's room, which, in Kitty's slow-moving dream, manifested itself as Fred Astaire languidly tap-dancing across the stage at the Palace Theatre to whisk her into his arms. 'Longthorne! I know you're in there.'

This was no song-and-dance routine, however. The urgency of her visitor's knocking snagged and punctured Kitty's heavy, dreamy sleep, leaking a trail of panic behind her sluggish thoughts.

'Kitty Longthorne! Answer the door, this instant!'

It was Matron.

The switch from deep sleep to wide awake was instant. Realisation that she was in trouble flooded the empty space in her mind, washing Fred Astaire away.

'Coming, matron!' Kitty threw her eiderdown off the bed. Her breath steamed on the icy air. She pulled off the chunky knitted hat she'd gone to bed in, smoothing her dishevelled hair. Stumbling, she stuffed her bed-sock-clad feet into Ned's old carpet slippers and shuffled in her heavy blanket-like man's dressing gown to the door. Would Matron give her a dressing down for her bed attire as well as for how she'd spoken to Sister Iris?

Saying a quick prayer for leniency, she opened the door.

Matron was standing before her, crisp and starched as

ever in her uniform but with a look of intense displeasure on her face. 'May I come in?'

'Of course! Sorry I didn't come to the door straight away. I'm on nights, as you know and—'

'I don't need to hear your excuses, young lady.' Matron strode over to the only chair in the room, by the dressing table, and removed the spent clothes that were piled on it. 'I'm all too aware of what shift and whose ward you're currently on.' She sat down heavily, casting a judgemental look around the room.

Kitty had a decision to make. Should she stand by the harsh words she'd spoken to Sister Iris or apologise and eat humble pie?

'Sit down, girl,' Matron said.

Perching gingerly on the edge of her bed, Kitty examined her short fingernails. She felt certain she was standing at a fork in the road of her career which was more likely to lead her to the labour exchange than to promotion.

'Now, do you want to tell me about this new contretemps with Sister Iris? It's not often my own sleep is interrupted by an outraged senior member of staff, but, this morning, I've had an apoplectic sister on my hands, accusing you of all sorts, including professional misconduct.'

Kitty swallowed hard, her heart sinking. How stupid she'd been to think she'd fought a moral war and that Iris had finally acquiesced.

'What do you have to say for yourself?'

She answered in the smallest of voices but forced herself to look Matron in the eye as she revealed all about the long-standing mistreatment of Lily by Sister Iris and about Kitty's chance involvement with the admission of Dora Mackie to an overburdened casualty department. 'She was in a terrible way, was Mrs Mackie, so I had her rushed down to the operating theatre for emergency surgery. Understandably, I was late for my shift, and Sister Iris lost her rag.'

'Kitty!' Matron curled her lip. 'Your turns of phrase leave something to be desired.'

'Sorry, matron.'

'Go on.'

Kitty went on to describe the rest of the events that had led to her most recent bout of defiance. '. . . I thought, there's Sister Iris, reading a book and eating a bacon butty, and there's me, like a mug—'

Matron nodded. 'You left early. You deliberately diso- beyed orders from your superior?'

Kitty felt her lips prickling with fear. 'I suppose so, but—'

'And you spoke to Sister Iris in a manner unbecoming of a nurse?'

'We're both grown women. I was just doing my job and doing it well! I wasn't the one sat with my feet up during an emergency. Matron, she complained about Dora Mackie's turn for the worse like it was an inconvenience. As though it was my fault, and poor Dora was—'

Almost balking when Matron stood suddenly, Kitty got to her feet and took two steps backwards, waiting to be given the sack.

'For now,' Matron said, 'you're off that ward.'

'But what about Dora?'

'Your colleagues are every bit as capable as you. Dora Mackie is no longer your concern. You'll work under the stewardship of Sister Matilda on maternity.'

'With Violet? On the day shift?'

'Is that a problem? I thought you two were friends.' Matron narrowed her eyes, as though she were intuiting what had come to pass between Kitty and Violet over the past two years.

Realising she was treading a very fine line, Kitty smiled and nodded. 'I can't tell you how much I appreciate this. I don't want you to think I'm a troublemaker.'

'One could argue that you are being exactly that, Longthorne. You are skating on very thin ice, girl.'

'I know how it looks, what with my family and that. And the Sister Iris and Nurse Schwartz thing. It's just –'

Matron sighed. 'Get your sleep, Kitty. You begin your new shift tomorrow. Steer clear of Sister Iris. Poking at the wound won't do either of you any good.'

'You don't think I'm lying, do you?' Kitty wondered momentarily if she *had* been in the wrong. Surely not!

Matron pursed her lips. Her body stiffened as though she were about to turn and leave. 'If you have a problem with a senior member of staff and that happens to be your immediate superior, you need to remember to come to *me* about it. It's not befitting of a girl at your level in the nursing staff to try to tackle matters by herself. I shouldn't need to remind you of the pecking order in a place like this, should I? If the established structure is challenged, the entire house of cards comes down, and our patients – they're relying on us to save their lives. A hospital staff must function like an army. Every man knows his job, knows his place and carries out his orders.'

Kitty shook her head, mentally waving goodbye to her promotion prospects. 'I did forget my place and I apologise. Truly.' She was suddenly quaking with cold – or perhaps shock.

'You're shivering, young lady,' Matron said. 'Get back to bed. Go on.'

Alone once again, uncomfortably perspiring yet still freezing beneath her eiderdown, Kitty lay awake for a full hour, agonising over her future and whether she'd said the correct thing to Matron. Eventually, though, exhaustion smothered her overheated brain and she slept.

Kitty woke as the wintry daylight had started to fail and another interminable Arctic evening had started to drape itself over Davyhulme, entombing the place in bitter cold and deep, silencing snow that seemed to slow time. She'd grown used to the nightshift. Despite still being bone-tired, she found herself getting out of bed and pouring too much of the treacly liquid from her Camp coffee bottle into her cup. Kidding herself that the chicory would give her the same caffeinated kick as the delicious real coffee at Kardomah, she sipped her barely palatable hot drink, gave herself a good strip-wash in a sink full of hot water, and piled on as many layers of clothing as possible to fend off the infernal chill.

Trudging over to the hospital, satisfied that Sister Iris wouldn't arrive for the new nightshift for another hour, Kitty made straight for Dora Mackie's bedside. She found her patient propped up in bed, still breathing oxygen through a mask with a length of tubing plugged into her chest, just beneath her armpit. Pinkish fluid drained down the tube into a glass bucket that stood on the floor. Her head was band-aged and her face a palette of bruising purples and greens.

Dora was alive. Better than that, she was awake.

She recognised Kitty immediately. 'Hello, angel,' she said, holding her hand out.

Taking a seat by her bedside, Kitty gently and fleet-ingly squeezed Dora's hand. 'I went to see your children,' she said. 'Don't worry. Your next-door neighbour is doing a cracking job with them! Though they really need some medical attention.'

Audibly sobbing behind her mask, Dora said, 'Jesus, Mary and Joseph, thank heavens my babies are being taken care of. Thank you. God bless you.'

'Dora, they all have hacking coughs. They've got some of the worst nits I've ever seen. They have to see a doctor, very soon. If your neighbour or a family member can bring them into the children's emergency—'

'Oh, my babies. I miss my babies.' Tears rolled over the elastic that held Dora's oxygen mask in place. She snatched it away from her face and groaned mournfully.

Kitty took a clean handkerchief from her handbag and dabbed at Dora's eyes. 'There, there! You'll see them soon enough if you keep making progress like this. What you need is a break away from all this.' She smiled at the battered and bed-ridden woman, thinking about what James might potentially be able to do for her, if only he could loosen some purse-strings among the hospital's benefactors.

'Right now, I'd give anything just to be tucked up in my little house with . . .'

Dora's words petered off as though flurries of snow and eddies of freezing wind had crept into the ward and whipped away her breath. It was, however, a far more sinister visitor that had snatched her voice.

A wall of a man was suddenly looming at the foot of the bed, as though the ominous ghost of Christmas future had abruptly appeared on the ward. Kitty eyed his well-worn donkey jacket with its shining leather shoulder patches and large, bulging patch pockets. He wore dark, paint-splattered trousers, baggy and threadbare at the knee. His enormous feet were encased in hob-nail boots. The leather over the toes had split, revealing steel beneath, as though his flesh covered a skeleton of unyielding metal. His ruddy, square-jawed face had perhaps been handsome once, with dark-lashed, green eyes that still startled and a shock of black hair that had only just begun to beat a retreat towards his crown. But this mountain of muscle and sinew, clad in hard man's clothing, now sported a crooked nose that bore testament to several well-aimed punches. His hands were red-raw and cracked at the knuckles. It gave the impression that he'd once been a noble Celt, who had trodden the Giant's Causeway underfoot as though it were no more than a fairy ring of fanciful toadstools: warrior king stock, now gone to seed. No more Saxon hordes to conquer. No more Wehrmacht to skewer with his bayonet. Only a half-starved woman and her toddlers to use as a punchbag for those ham-like fists. Kitty shuddered and moved her chair backwards by an inch or two.

'Dora,' he said in a voice that was higher and softer than it should have been for a man of his stature. He reached into his pocket and brought out a small package wrapped in brown paper.

Dora's breathing had started to quicken. Kitty could sense from the way her body was rigid that she was in fear for her life.

'Francis.' Her voice cracked. 'I didn't think you'd come.'

Mr Mackie took a step towards the bed, looking expectantly at Kitty, as though it was her cue to leave Dora's bedside.

'Why on earth would I leave my Mrs in hospital, alone in a cold, hard bed? Sure, you're surrounded by handsome doctors and lovely young nurses, but they're no replacement for a husband's care, Dora. And the babies need you.'

Kitty remained seated in the chair by Dora's bedside, wondering what to do. Dora's breathing was shallow, her body tense. As the giant took another two steps towards her, holding out her gift, Dora started to weep silently; struggling to catch her breath.

'I bought you a comb for your beautiful hair,' Mackie said, unwrapping the cheap gift with one hand and pulling Dora's mask off with another. 'Let me see you.' He grabbed her chin roughly and yanked Dora's face to one side, studying his purple and green handiwork.

'That's enough, sir! Can I kindly ask you to step away?' Kitty said, rising to her feet, speaking as loud as she could so that the other nurses could hear there was a problem.

She snatched the mask off Mackie and tried to replace it around Dora's nose and mouth. 'I'm Dora's nurse and she's very, *very* poorly, so if you'd just—'

'Cheeky little hussy! Don't you be telling me how to be around my own wife!' Mackie shouted.

By the time Kitty realised that the whistling noise was his raised hand sweeping through the air towards her head, it was too late.

Chapter 28

'Help!' Kitty shouted, as the impact from Mackie's blow knocked her to the floor. 'Help me!'

'That'll teach you!' Mackie said, standing over her with flaring nostrils and a look of satisfaction on his face.

Amid the startled yelps and concerned shouting from the patients who were watching the attack, Kitty heard a man's voice cut through the commotion.

'I say, sir! How dare you? Yes, you! I'm talking to you, you brute.'

She looked up to find Richard Collins rolling up the sleeves of his white coat, squaring up to Mackie.

Mackie, at least six inches taller than the anaesthetist, laughed raucously. 'Shove your gallantry, you berk. I was leaving anyway.' He pushed past Richard with such force that Richard was knocked into a folding screen that went clattering to the floor.

With flame-red cheeks, looking utterly flustered, the anaesthetist seemed to regain his composure and offered his hand to Kitty. 'My dear, are you quite all right?'

Kitty got to her feet. Her first thoughts were for poor Dora, who was gasping for breath with no oxygen mask on. 'I'm fine! Thank you. I'm fine!' She waved him away and tended to her distressed patient, adjusting Dora's oxygen supply and smoothing her brow. 'Dr Collins, just make sure that brute doesn't come back!' At the entrance to the ward, however, she could hear Mackie barking at another man.

'Get out of the bloody way, you little jumped-up arsehole!'

Mackie's second challenger sounded unperturbed. 'The police are on their way. If you think you can take a swing at me in the meantime, sir, I encourage you to try.'

It was James! Kitty craned her neck to see the surgeon standing perfectly straight in front of Mackie, arms beside him, looking completely unperturbed. Mackie took a swing at him and in a blur of sudden movement, James seemed to grab hold of the man-mountain's fist and twist him around and onto the floor as though he were nothing sturdier than a rag doll. Now, James was sitting astride the giant, holding his arms behind his back.

'You do *not* assault our staff, Mr Mackie,' James said. 'Yes. I know your name!'

Mackie tried to look round to lock eyes with his surprise assailant. He shouted a string of curses that made the nurses standing nearby gasp and tut.

James allowed Mackie to get to his feet, though he held his arms behind his back in what appeared to be a painful lock.

When Kitty was satisfied that Dora's breathing had calmed, she left her side to join the motley band that was gathering at the entrance to the ward. Clutching her battered jaw, she pointed to Mackie.

'This man just punched me,' she told the onlookers. 'He's the husband of one of our patients – Mrs Mackie. Given his left hook, I'd say it's less likely that a tumble down the stairs knocked hell's bells out of Mrs Mackie and more likely that she was beaten to death's door by this monstrosity of a man.'

'Shut your trap, you silly, interfering cow.' Mackie was seemingly unrepentant, struggling hard against James's grip.

'That's quite enough from you, you oik!' Richard exclaimed. 'Let's get him down to the foyer, Dr Williams. The police can take him from there.'

Mackie took a step towards Richard, straining and finally breaking free of James. 'You? *You* tell me what to do and where to go, you ponce? I'd like to see it. I bet you didn't even fight in the war, did you? You Nancy boys in your white coats are all the same! Lily-livered, like the French!'

Richard simply smiled and coolly withdrew a syringe from his white-coat pocket. He unsheathed the needle. Kitty could see that the barrel was empty, but Mackie didn't know that.

'Unfortunately for you, Mr Mackie, I'm an anaesthetist. You can come calmly, or would you prefer I sedated you?'

'You wouldn't dare!'

'Try me.'

Richard lunged forward quickly so that he'd pressed the needle of the empty syringe against Mackie's chest before the crazed wife-beater could lash out and knock it from him. Clearly flustered, Mackie paused long enough for James to renew his grip on the behemoth's upper arms.

As the men strong-armed Mackie away, Kitty and James exchanged a glance. Kitty knew, at that moment, that he fully understood the plight of Dora Mackie and her children. Mackie's strength and aggression were constantly a threat, and her murder was only one tantrum away.

Left alone, Kitty clutched at her aching face, wondering at the ludicrous turn of events in the last forty-eight hours. She was poised to return to Dora's bedside but spotted Sister Iris, padding down the corridor to begin her shift.

With a thundering heartbeat, Kitty darted out of sight behind a wheeled screen that had handily been left just outside the entrance to the ward. She prayed silently that Iris would not spot her feet peeping out beneath the steel frame. The last thing she needed was another confrontation with the contrary sister, who would almost certainly somehow manage to blame her for Mackie's misdemeanours.

Making good her getaway, once Iris had pushed through the ward doors and out of sight, Kitty's pulse didn't slow until she was back in the freezing cold foyer.

The place was hopping, not with the normal swarm of patients and doctors, hastening to their next appointment or emergency, but with three police constables – two who were bundling a handcuffed Mackie into the back of a waiting Black Maria police van, and one who was taking statements in his notebook from Richard and James.

Richard was deep in conversation with the constable, with James chipping in.

Not wishing to interrupt, Kitty kept her head down and scurried past an elderly man being pushed in a wheelchair by a young woman. She'd almost made it beyond the Black Maria, the doors of which were now being slammed shut, when she felt a warm hand on her cold shoulder.

'Kitty!'

She turned around to find James looking at her with undisguised concern etched on his handsome face. The skin on his wrists – just visible inside the cuffs of his suit jacket – was puckered up with goose bumps; the hairs standing on end.

'Go back inside!' she said. 'You'll catch your death out here, and then where will we be?'

He reached out and gently touched the place where Mackie's hand had caught her jaw. 'It's bruising. You should take some arnica. Does it hurt?'

'I've put ice on it already,' Kitty lied. She wanted to tell him that it did hurt, but not quite so much as the feel of his fingertips on her face. To be touched by the man she'd loved all these years, who had opted to give his caresses to Violet in her stead, hurt more than any hard slap from a stranger. Instinctively, she put her hand on top of his fleetingly but then took a step back, breaking the contact. 'I'll be fine. But now you can see what Dora's up against. Imagine being laid up on a ward when your tiny children are coughing their guts up in dire conditions, at the mercy of an ogre like Mackie.'

James was looking at her intently. Regret seemed to form dull cataracts over his normally glowing brown eyes.

'I spend my life trying to fix the symptoms,' he said. 'Maybe I *should* look harder at the root causes. Though I'm not sure I have the aptitude for that level of empathy. My strengths lie in a level head, a steady hand and a strong stomach.' He chuckled and quaked as a flurry of snow whipped around his legs. His breath steamed on the air.

Was Kitty merely imagining there was more to his wistful expression than just the biting cold? It didn't matter. He belonged to Violet. He'd made his choice.

'You're a powerful man in this hospital, James. See what you can do.'

'Why do you care so much?' he asked unexpectedly. 'I mean, about Dora?'

Kitty cast a contemplative glance at the Black Maria and frowned quizzically. 'It'd be easy for a girl like me to become a woman like her.' She cleared her throat, thinking briefly of her mother and how history repeated itself. 'Now, go back inside! Go on! The great Dr Williams is no good to us as an icicle.'

*

As she trudged back towards the nurses' home to get some more rest in preparation for the new maternity ward day shift that would begin tomorrow, she almost slipped on the icy path when the bells of an ambulance started to ring.

The ambulance tore past her, spattering her legs with freezing slush.

'Cobblers,' she said under her breath as the icy water bit into her skin. 'Damn this never-ending winter.'

Suddenly, the din of another ambulance struck up, too loud in the muffled hush of the falling snow. It pulled out of a bay by the entrance to casualty, revving its engines. What on earth was going on? Kitty wondered.

Three nurses were suddenly running towards her, somewhat gingerly on the slippery path.

'Get your uniform on!' one of them told Kitty. 'Matron wants all hands on deck.'

'What's happened?'

Her colleagues had already shot past her.

One turned around, clutching her nurse's cap to her head, and yelled, 'They found an unexploded bomb. There's been a terrible accident.'

Chapter 29

When Kitty arrived in casualty, the place was already teeming with the injured and the bloodied, thanks to the infernal icy conditions. One of the longest-serving ward sisters was giving a briefing in the office. Standing on the sidelines in the cramped, packed room, Kitty spied Violet and waved to her, resolving to be as friendly as they'd ever been and to ignore the ache in her heart. She edged her way through the throng of nursing staff until she was standing by Violet's side.

'What's all this, then?' she whispered just loud enough for Violet to hear.

'Gangsters!' Violet said breathily with undisguised excitement seeming to light up her freckles. 'Long story.'

'Are you paying attention, you two?' the sister asked. She was a tiny but stern woman whom everyone knew to have worked at the hospital since its opening in 1929. She spoke with the authority of someone who didn't suffer fools at all, let alone gladly.

'Sorry, Sister Gladys,' Kitty said.

Violet merely smiled. 'It's all just so dramatic!'

'What is?' Sister Gladys said, narrowing her eyes at Violet. 'The prospect of scores of men with head injuries and crushed limbs being brought in here? Or the danger of an unexploded Satan bomb that could kill hundreds being uncovered in a derelict Stretford bakery? Which one of those little dramas entertains you the most, Jones?'

The smile slid from Violet's face. 'I just meant —' She fell silent and looked down at her glittering engagement ring.

When the briefing had finished, Kitty started to gather from the stockroom the dressings, cotton wool and other accoutrements she would need when the casualties started to arrive.

Violet came in and snatched her assembled pile out of her hands. 'Thanks for putting these together. You've saved me a job!' She winked.

'I wasn't—'

'So, Molly Bickerstaff took the call from the fire service,' Violet said, gabbling away conspiratorially. 'Pass me some more bandages, there's a darling. And she said that the bomb was found when a group of local gangsters — they've been using the disused bakery as their headquarters! Can you *imagine*?' Her azure blue eyes widened. She was like a giddy child who had just spotted an unguarded bowl of sweets. 'Anyway, these gangsters were moving a printing press, of all things, into the bakery. It was apparently so heavy and it was so dark in there that they lost their footing and the whole caboodle fell through a big hole in the floor. But it wasn't just an ordinary cellar. It was a pit of about twenty feet that had been left by a *colossal bomb*.'

'How come nobody knew about it?' Kitty asked, gathering her materials anew.

Violet shrugged. 'How would I know? I think the place was abandoned after the Blitz because it was in such dangerous shape. My guess is the owners wrote the place off without realising the hole in the roof and the floor had been made by a Satan bomb. Imagine!'

'What were they hoping to print? Any idea?'

'Molly Bickerstaff thinks they're counterfeiters. I suppose we'll know more when the police interrogate the men. *If* any of them survive! Imagine if the bomb goes off . . .' She took a sharp breath. 'Imagine if there's an explosion while the ambulance men are trying to get the gangsters onto stretchers. Ooh, this will be in the *Manchester Evening News*, make no mistake.' Then her slender eyebrows knitted together and her freckled brow furrowed. 'I hope James didn't accompany any of the ambulances.' She bit her lip. 'It's just the sort of silly, selfless thing he'd do.'

'Did he know about the call?' Kitty conjured the memory of James standing on the icy path with her, touching her jaw. She touched the place where Mackie had slapped her. It was tender. 'I was talking to him about a patient just before the ambulances started to leave. Moments before.'

'I'm not James Williams's secretary. I have no idea where he is from one day to the next. He's so obsessed with his work, I'm lucky to see him once in a blue moon at the moment.'

If James had accompanied the ambulances to the bomb site, Violent seemed blithely indifferent to the risk he may have taken. But Kitty wasn't. She left the storeroom and found Sister Gladys.

'Which doctors have been drafted in to help?' she asked.

Sister Gladys, who was taking blood from an elderly lady in a side cubicle, scowled at Kitty over the top of her pearl-winged glasses. 'The ones who were on site. Professor Baird-Murray, Mr Galbraith, Dr Williams.'

Feeling the blood drain from her cheeks, Kitty swallowed hard. 'None of the doctors went to the scene of the accident, did they?'

'I believe brave Dr Williams volunteered, in case there were injuries that needed dealing with on the spot. They're sending the military in to diffuse the bomb, I hear. Dangerous business.'

'Oh.' Kitty felt the walls of the cubicle begin to sway.

'Are you quite all right, Longthorne?' Sister Gladys was talking to Kitty though her voice seemed like it was coming from the bottom of a pond. She grabbed Kitty's forearm to steady her. For a small woman, her grip was deadly.

'I'm fine. I just haven't slept much since my last shift.'

'Then get a drink of water and get on with it, girl. That bomb in Stretford doesn't know that the war's over. This is no time for self-indulgence.'

Kitty staggered away to deal with a bedpan from one of the existing admissions. She thought about the possibility of James being blown to smithereens. There was so much she'd never told him that she still wanted to say. She couldn't imagine a world without him. And yet, it was Violet who stood to lose a fiancé if things went awry. Should she tell her friend? Oblivious and smiling, Violet was tending to a young boy who had broken his arm in a fall on an icy lane. No. Kitty couldn't worry her unnecessarily. And yet, wouldn't she want to know if her beloved was in danger? Did Kitty have the right to withhold such important information from her friend?

'Violet.'

'Yes?'

'Sister Gladys said Dr Williams hopped on one of the ambulances. He's gone to the scene in case somebody needs immediate attention.'

Violet stood up and looked blankly at Kitty. If she was concerned, it didn't show in her face. She smiled warmly. 'So brave! Aren't I a lucky gal?' Then she stooped to tie a sling for the boy.

Blinking hard, Kitty wondered that Violet was seemingly unperturbed by the news that the man she hoped to marry was within spitting distance of one of the Luftwaffe's most powerful bombs. Did she not love James?

Reflecting on how undeserving of James's devotion Violet was and how painful unrequited love could be, Kitty forced herself to remain as alert and professional as she possibly could, treating the backlog of people in the waiting room until the disastrous cases came in from the bakery. When they did come, they were in terrible shape, with crushed arms and legs; caked in gore from head injuries and the dust of falling masonry. She looked for James among the arrivals but couldn't spot him.

"Ey up, love!' an ambulance driver said to her, as he and another man wheeled a rattling trolley through the casualty entrance doors. 'This one's in a bad way. Stuck under a printing press, would you believe it? Bet that leg'll come off.'

The screaming patient strapped to the trolley looked familiar to her. He was dark haired with a stubbled chin and appeared to be in his forties. He had a distinctive scar on his left eyebrow and a pierced ear like a merchant sailor. Where had Kitty seen him before? It would come to her.

'Was Dr Williams there when you rescued this man?' she asked.

'Aye,' the driver said. 'He was the one what put the tourniquet on this feller when he came out from under that printer. Big heavy thing it is. Like what you get in the Express building. Christ knows what they were doing with it in a derelict bakery. Poor Dr Williams.'

'What do you mean, "*Poor* Dr Williams"? Is he hurt?'

The ambulance driver looked at her askance and began to shake his head ruefully. 'Haven't you heard?'

'Heard *what*?'

Chapter 30

The ambulance driver leaned in towards Kitty, speaking with a conspiratorial air. 'Every second that ticks by is bringing Dr Williams closer to death. You mark my words. That bomb what he's sitting on – I had a good look down the hole. Thirty feet deep, it must have been. I've never seen anything like it. It were bigger than the Lord Mayor's front parlour. No word of a lie. Big as a bloody fire engine. How they didn't realise it were down there, I'll never know. And what there was in Stretford to warrant dropping it, your guess is as good as mine, love. The army feller said if it goes off, that's the end of the errand for miles around. He was a cockney, mind.' He curled his lip.

With a privately quailing heart as she marched alongside the trolley, Kitty led the paramedics to Professor Baird-Murray. The professor was wearing a white gown and mask, ready for surgery.

'You, young lady!' Baird-Murray said to Kitty. 'Fanny, or whatever you're called.'

'It's Kitty, professor. Kitty Longthorne.'

'Quite. Look, Fanny, we're dreadfully understaffed and you're a safe pair of hands, aren't you? Scrub up, dear girl, and assist me!'

Kitty nodded and immediately made her way to the sink and started to scrub her hands and forearms under the scalding tap. Within minutes, she was handing the professor a pair of shears with which he removed the patient's trousers. Dark, viscous blood oozed from a shocking wound to the thigh – what was left of it. Kitty had seen many a similarly bad wound on the US soldiers she had treated. Shrapnel, gunshot and burns had left thousands of young men crippled or disfigured for life. So, when Baird-Murray said the leg would have to come off, Kitty was hardly surprised.

The anaesthetist, whom Kitty hadn't noticed earlier, as he'd been standing with his back to her, turned around.

'Ready?' It was Richard. Even though the bottom half of his face was covered by his mask, Kitty could tell he was smiling.

She forced a smile back, though her new admirer was the last person she'd hoped to see in an emergency surgery when her thoughts were elsewhere.

Within moments of Richard's ministrations, the patient was under.

Making careful preparations to stem the blood-flow, Kitty handed Baird-Murray the saw, and the amputation of the unsalvageable lower leg was underway. It was halfway through the procedure when Kitty realised that she recognised the patient from one of her father's illicit card games in their old back parlour, before the war.

'Is this man's name Fred Smethwick?' Kitty asked.

'I haven't a clue!' Baird-Murray said. 'No distractions please, Fanny. Scalpel!'

With the operation concluded successfully, Kitty tracked down the man's effects, which had been left in Violet's care.

'Have you checked the pockets, Vi?'

'Why would I?' Violet said, smiling and wrinkling her nose. 'They're nothing but smelly old rags.'

'The contents of a man's pockets can be revealing.' Kitty felt her way around the man's jacket and happened upon a promising lump in the inside pocket. She pulled out a battered old wallet, stuffed with twenty pounds. She gasped.

'My word!' Violet said.

'A king's ransom!' Kitty stared at the money, reasoning that this was as much as she earned in a full year. 'But what's this?' She leafed through the other papers in the wallet. There were more in a tightly bound bundle – or rather in a book – stashed in the man's inside pocket of his tailored jacket. 'Coupons?' Staring at the coupons, Kitty could see that they weren't exactly like the familiar tokens in her mother's coupon book that she used weekly to obtain her rations. They neither felt right nor looked right. Oh so similar, but not the same. Then Kitty realised what she saw. These were counterfeit coupons.

She was just wondering whether or not she should share her discovery with Violet when Sister Gladys popped her head around the door.

'Ah, there you are, Longthorne. I have a job for you. Hop in the ambulance, there's a dear. Dr Williams needs help at the accident site and he's requested you.'

Kitty blushed. Violet's face was thunderous. But the sense of urgency swept away any chance of a confrontation.

'Chop, chop, Longthorne!' Sister Gladys said, clapping her hands. 'This is no time for dilly-dallying!'

'I'm not frightened,' Kitty told the ambulance driver. 'It'll take more than an unexploded bomb to scare me!' She swallowed hard and clutched at the corners of her nurse's cape as they almost slid along the icy road to Stretford.

Skidding to a halt, Kitty hopped out with a thundering heartbeat, so anxious that she was in such close proximity to mortal danger and so exhilarated to have been requested by James that she didn't even feel the cold.

The military had cordoned off the area at least two hundred yards beyond the bakery. Kitty felt like she was entering the frontline of the war that had been won two years earlier. With some trepidation, she approached a soldier.

'I'm here to assist the doctor,' she said. Her medical bag was heavy, loaded with the various instruments that James had requested via the ambulance driver.

The soldier nodded and lifted the cordon.

Several decaying Victorian buildings comprised a row of shops. They were covered in thick slabs of forgetful snow, like royal icing hiding the truth of a disappointing cake. A car was parked outside a grocery. A bicycle had been left beneath the awning of a barber shop. The only signs of life in this land-locked rendition of the *Marie Celeste* came from a bakery that stood alone like a ghostly mausoleum. Green-uniformed soldiers stood, passing large chunks of masonry and splintered timbers along a line.

'This way, nurse!' one of the lads said, ushering her into the building. 'The doctor's waiting. Mind how you go!'

Immediately outside the bakery were two oblong forms on stretchers, covered with green army blankets. Clearly, not everyone had been rescued from this criminal calamity.

Inside had been temporarily lit by large, portable field lights on tripods. There were the remnants of a shop front with shelves. On a counter thick with dust, there was an old till and weighing scales wrapped in cobwebs. They looked as though they had been abandoned on the day that the

Luftwaffe had paid a fateful visit to the row of shops, forever waiting in vain for customers to return. The place felt sad. Out back, however, was even worse. Beyond the old ovens was a cavernous double-height space. There was a large hole in the roof above that marked where the bomb had come through, but the place was lit by bright emergency lamps. They shone on a scene of devastation, where the printing press had fallen into a deep pit.

Tentatively, Kitty approached the edge. She looked some twenty or thirty feet down into the pit to see James standing on top of a pile of rubble that barely covered the largest bomb she had ever seen. He was busy about an injured man who was covered in blood and trapped beneath the giant press. Looking up, his taut face seemed to relax somewhat.

'Excellent! There you are,' he said. 'Get one of the soldiers to hoist you down. We have to work quickly.'

'I brought the bag.' Kitty waved the medical kit but James had already turned back to the patient. She eyed the bomb warily. Two men – presumably explosives experts – were leaning into the pit, examining it. What choice did she have but to clamber down and help?

A soldier tied a harness around Kitty and lowered her to the mound of rubble. She opened the medical bag, which contained several scalpels, anaesthetic and a saw.

'The printing press just won't budge,' James explained. 'I'm going to have to do the amputation here and now, else this gentleman won't make it. As it is, I think he has a broken back.'

Kitty nodded, perching precariously on a large timber. She glanced at the unconscious man whose head was entirely bloodied and covered in masonry dust. The contours of his face, however, could not be obscured. She gasped.

'Oh,' she said, suddenly dizzy. 'Sweet Jesus!' The man who had a Satan bomb for a bed and a printing press for a blanket was none other than Kitty's father. She wanted to shout, 'Dad!' but bit her tongue. The police were waiting outside to cuff any of the surviving injured, whether they were walking wounded or hospital-bound.

James looked up at her. He lowered his voice to a whisper. 'Yes. I'm sorry. He's aged a lot, but his eyebrows and that distinctive mole on the side of his nose – I recognised him straight away from the photograph you showed me in Windermere.'

Kitty was revisited by the bitter-sweet memory of that trip to the Lake District with James. It had turned out to be their last date before his interest had mysteriously waned and Violet had edged into the frame. Before the Nazis had blasted away the optimism of Britain, she'd sat on a blanket by the shores of a sunny Lake Windermere, reached into her handbag, and had plucked a photo from between the pages of her diary. She'd shown her new beau the formal posed portrait of her family that had been taken on her parents' fifteenth wedding anniversary – the second of only two remaining family photographs that had miraculously survived, thanks to the sturdy old wooden sideboard that had confounded the Luftwaffe's best efforts. To fourteen-year-old Kitty, her father had looked like a toff in borrowed finery, but James had presumably seen Bert Longthorne for the working-class underachiever that he was. Had that been the beginning of the end for them? Had the barrister's son decided that day that he shouldn't stoop to conquer a poor girl's heart after all?

'It's a conflict of interest and the last thing I want is to put you in harm's way,' James went on, oblivious to her inner turmoil. 'But I thought, given the circumstances, you'd better be the one to assist me.'

Staring at her father, for all she loathed him, it pained her to see him fighting for his life, with his arm trapped beneath two tons of metal. Kitty needed to focus on the task in hand. 'What do you need me to do?'

'I've tied his arm with a tourniquet already,' James said. 'Let's clean the area up, and I'll get cracking. The sooner we're away from this bomb, the better. The army chaps said it's unstable.'

'If you wish long enough, wish strong enough, you will come to know, wishing will make it so'. In her head, Kitty repeated the line from the Glen Miller song throughout the messy and brutal procedure. Repetition and focussing on a happy thought was the only way she was going to get through this calmly. She tried not to think of the man whose arm James was sawing off as her father. She pushed away all thoughts of the Black Maria police vans waiting outside the cordon and the unexploded bomb that could blow them all to kingdom come at any moment.

'Have the police said anything about what was going on here?' she whispered as James sutured what was left of her father's left arm.

He shook his head. 'There are boxes and boxes stacked in a corner and loose sheets printed with coupons scattered all over the floor. I noticed them when I arrived. You couldn't miss them. I'm not saying your father's a criminal, but—'

'I'm well aware of my father's pedigree,' Kitty said sourly.

'I'm sorry. I didn't mean to judge. I would never—'

'You already did. You made it very clear two years ago that I wasn't good enough for you. Now, kindly drop the subject, please.' She felt tears prickling at the backs of her eyes.

Out of the corner of her eye, she could see James glance up from his careful stitching and look at her askance. He opened his mouth to speak, seemed to think better of it, and merely shook his head.

There was a sudden creaking sound of metal moving and an ominous clank. The bomb beneath them shifted by several inches.

Chapter 31

'We're running out of time. Here,' one of the explosives experts said, blanching at the cloud of dust that the sudden slip had kicked up, 'I need this printing press out of the way so I can diffuse that bomb, else they'll be dropping bits of us off at Southern Cemetery, never mind the hospital.'

'Lower the stretcher,' James said to one of the soldiers above. He sounded hoarse and weary.

Though they worked together to slide the stretcher beneath her father without causing further injury to his back or neck, James didn't look at Kitty. It didn't matter, though. The sight of her father with a bandaged stump, covered in blood and masonry dust in that pit blocked out all other salient thought. For years she'd hated him and wished him dead for the shame he'd brought on her family and the hardship her mother had had to endure because of his criminal ways. Now, he might yet die or be paralysed for life. That blow to the head looked serious. Was there any point in saying that she loved him in spite of all his flaws?

As the soldiers lifted her father up out of the pit, Kitty started to weep silently, wiping her tears on her cape. James noticed and put his arm around her.

'We'll do our best for him.'

She pulled away. His words were empty. There was never even the suggestion of an apology.

The harness dropped down and Kitty allowed herself to be hoisted up to fresher air. Still, when she peered through a veil of tears back down into the pit, she couldn't help but meet James's gaze and pray he too made it back up safely.

'Thanks, chaps,' he said, reaching the top and being pulled back onto a stable patch of flooring.

'You get yourself gone quickly, doctor,' one of the soldiers said. 'You've been a right hero down there. But now it's time to leave it to us.'

Together, Kitty and James walked briskly to the ambulance and, in silence, clambered into the back to sit with her father.

Kitty could feel words of love and regret and sorrow fermenting inside her. Tension thrummed in the air inside that ambulance as it skidded and slid its way clear of the cordoned-off area.

James reached out and took her hand. She tried to pull it away.

'Here, stop tormenting me, for pity's sake!' Kitty glanced over at her father but he was strapped to the trolley and hooked up to a saline drip, out cold.

James held on to her hand firmly and stroked her knuckles. The sinew in his jaw flinched and he stared solemnly at her shoulder, as if looking her in the eye was too difficult. 'Kitty, I—' He exhaled deeply, opened his mouth again, but nothing came out.

'You what? What, James? Are you about to say something you'd say in front of Violet? Or are you about to make some grand revelation that you think will compensate for two years of misery, watching you run off with my so-called best friend, when I thought you had serious intentions towards me? Or am I presuming too much, thinking that a fine doctor like you – a barrister's son – might still harbour feelings for the small, plain girl with a big heart that he left for dust?' Kitty felt so exhausted by all that had happened that she was too tired to man her internal defences. The walls seemed to crumble to allow the hurt to scramble over and escape. 'I'm sorry that I don't have silk dresses and wear make-up and flirt with every man that looks my way. I'm sorry my mother isn't a socialite and that I don't have nicely turned ankles. I'm sorry that you thought all of those things were important. I hope you're happy with your choice, James, because that is what you chose. You picked a vain girl with money because she'd look nice on your arm and would keep your family happy. I might just be from a two-up-two-down in Hulme with a father who's bent as a nine-bob note, James Williams, but I know a thing or two about how the world works.' Finally, Kitty felt as though she'd extinguished the fire within her.

The ambulance was approaching the snow-covered clock tower of Park Hospital, slowing to a standstill with fresh snow crunching and squeaking beneath the tyres. James looked forlornly at her. A solitary tear ran onto his cheek and his Adam's apple rose and fell inside his dirt-streaked neck.

'I never stopped loving you, Kitty, and I don't know what to do about it. It hurts every day. I'm sorry. Is there a way I—?'

'You pick your flipping moments, don't you?' Kitty said, trying and failing to digest what he'd finally revealed of his feelings. She held her hands up. 'James, just stop! I can't be doing with this, right now. Do me a favour. Just save my dad – for my mam's sake, if nothing else.'

She watched as her father's trolley was pulled out of the ambulance and followed as he was wheeled through the insistent snow that had settled, despite the salt on the path. James accompanied her in silence. Before they reached the doors and the prying eyes of the other hospital staff, he slipped his warm hand around hers and squeezed gently.

'I'll do my best for him, Kitty. I promise.' James let go and turned to the ambulance drivers. 'Gentlemen, kindly wheel the patient straight to X-ray. I'm deeply concerned about that gash to his head and potential spinal injury. Tell the radiologist it's of the utmost importance that . . .'

While he was facing the other way, briefing the men, Kitty felt a desperate need to slip away. Her head was pounding and her heart aching with the enormity of her father's accident and James's confession. Blinking away her tears, she spied two police constables, waiting with the handcuffed men from the bakery. Could these be her father's accomplices?

Leaving James to call after her in vain, Kitty made a beeline for the officers. She lowered her voice and spoke into the ear of the more senior-looking man.

'Can I have a word, please?'

He nodded. 'What is it, love?'

'I've just come from the bakery myself,' she said. 'Assisting the surgeon who attended the scene. I see these men are cuffed and I noticed a couple of officers carrying boxes out of the place. If you don't mind me asking, what's been going on?' She tried to smile and look winsome, batting her lashes as she'd seen Violet do, whenever she'd wanted something from a man.

The constable looked down at her. He seemed so tall and slightly forbidding in his dark uniform and bobby's helmet. 'I'm afraid I can't discuss that sort of thing with you, love.'

'But these are criminals I'm having to treat, aren't they?' she whispered, glancing pointedly at the cuffed patient, who was writhing in apparent agony in his chair, cursing and shouting about wrongful arrest and miscarriage of justice. 'I'm just worried for my own and my fellow nurses' safety, officer. Is it true, they're dangerous gangsters?'

Looking down at his gleaming black boots, the constable chewed the inside of his cheek. 'I shouldn't be telling you any of this,' he said quietly, 'but yes. It's a notorious counterfeiting ring.' He grinned widely. The day had clearly been a roaring success for the police, at least. 'Coupons. We've been after them for months. But don't worry, love. I don't think they'll start swinging punches at you.'

'Will they all go to prison?'

'The ones we caught. Aye.'

Kitty nodded and forced a smile. If her father survived, he'd go back to Strangeways. That wasn't the worst possible outcome, she calculated, given the tyranny of his reign at home. Something the bobby had said, however, piqued her curiosity. The ones we caught. Kitty wondered about her brother Ned. Was it possible that he'd been involved in the coupon swindle?

She made a mental note to keep a watchful eye on Ned's activity and wondered if he'd dare come to visit their father in hospital. If he stayed away, surely that was a sign he'd been one of the culprits who had fled. Or would Ned be brazen enough to show up regardless? It frustrated her that she never quite had the measure of her twin. She desperately wanted Ned to be better than the bad reputation that dogged the Longthorne men.

Deciding that her priority was to slip out and convey the dreadful news to her mother, Kitty glanced around casualty.

There was such pandemonium with the sudden influx of injured men, that surely she wouldn't be missed for just a quarter of an hour.

Stealthily leaving casualty through a side door, she trudged and skidded out of the snow-bound hospital site and shivered her way to the local post office before it shut. Handing over her money, she sent a telegram relaying the dreaded news to her mother:

Mam STOP Dad has been in terrible accident STOP Please come to Park Hospital straight away STOP Kitty

Chapter 32

'Kitty! There you are!' Violet said as Kitty emerged from the bathroom.

At 5.30 a.m., the nurses' home was so cold, crystalline florets of ice were forming on the insides of the windows. Kitty's teeth clacked as she clutched at her damp towel and held her ugly dressing gown closed against the chill. Her woollen hat was pulled low over her ears.

'Morning, Vi. First time on a ward together in quite some time, eh? See you downstairs in half an hour?'

Kitty tried to push past her friend, but Violet had other ideas.

'Darling, you're *not* sleeping in a knitted hat and a man's dressing gown, are you?' she asked, eyeing Kitty's bed attire. She looked down at Kitty's bed-sock-clad feet and curled her lip.

Violet's own shining red hair was already immaculately coiffed and her ginger eyelashes had been carefully darkened with soot or perhaps even proper mascara.

'Is that *rouge* you're wearing?' Kitty asked.

'That's not all!' Violet giggled conspiratorially. She held her hand beneath her chin as though posing for a photographer. 'James bought me some Helena Rubenstein foundation. It's all the go, *if* you can afford it. What do you think?'

News of the expensive gift from James rankled with Kitty. She calculated that her friend must have been up at four to be looking so groomed at such an ungodly hour. 'Matron's going to spot it and you'll be for the high jump. She'll make you scrub it off.'

'Oh, Kitty. You really must make more of yourself or you'll never get a husband,' Violet said.

'I've got more to worry about than looking like a Hollywood actress.'

'But darling, you could look like Veronica Lake, if you made an effort. Let me help you! We need to cover up that bruise, for a start. Blimey, Kitty! Have your patients been beating you?'

Kitty had almost forgotten about the right hook from Mackie. She touched the tender place on her jaw and winced. 'Violet, we're about to start a shift on the maternity ward in the worst winter in living memory or whatever it is the papers are claiming. There're icicles like carrots hanging from the rafters. My dad's lost his arm and God alone knows what shape his spine is in. Really, pack it in!'

'Ooh! Aren't you prickly?' Violet's smile fell from her tinted lips – almost certainly enhanced with more than just a dab of petroleum jelly. 'And I thought us working together would be a gas.'

'It will be. I'm really looking forward to it. There's just a lot going on.'

Kitty knew she had to make this new arrangement work. Matron had given her a second chance and was depending on her to toe the line. It wasn't going to be easy, though. There was the small issue of James confessing that he still harboured love for Kitty, which left a large question mark hanging over his engagement to Violet.

Against her will, a small smile tugged at the corners of Kitty's mouth.

'Ah. There we go,' Violet said in far-too-loud a voice for the hour. She clicked her fingers. 'That's more like it! Now, all you need is to do away with the tea-cosy on your head and the revolting dressing gown. We can't have you turning the labouring mothers to stone, can we?'

'Look, Vi. I'll see you at the start of our shift. I've got things I need to do beforehand.'

Violet raised an eyebrow. 'Shall I save you some breakfast?'

Kitty shook her head. 'It's kind of you, but honestly, I'll sort myself out. I'll see you on the ward.'

She left her crestfallen colleague standing in the freezing hallway and repaired to her room.

Dressing quickly, Kitty made her way over to the hospital. Her first stop was her father's bedside. He was on a ward with other men, where the sound of snoring ricocheted off the distempered walls and high ceilings. At that time in the morning, the lights were still low and the nightshift nurses kept a watchful eye on their charges from a desk at the head of the ward.

Bert Longthorne's bed was immediately marked out by the policeman who was nodding off in the chair next to him.

As Kitty padded softly down towards her father, it was clear that his good hand was cuffed to the bedframe. His head had been bandaged and he'd been hooked up to a drip. Drawing close, she realised he was out cold. Was it a natural slumber or was he still unconscious? His notes at the foot of the bed revealed little. Kitty scanned the page, covered in figures and scribbled observations, but could see nothing of his X-ray results. Had James been back to see him at all?

'Have Bert Longthorne's X-rays come back yet?' she whispered to the nurses on duty.

Her colleagues shrugged.

'Dr Williams came to check on him in the night. Said to treat him as a spinal injury.' the older nurse said. 'You'll have to ask him yourself when he does his rounds.'

'Is he a relation of yours?' the younger nurse said. 'Your surname's Longthorne, isn't it?'

Kitty blushed, leaning on the desk with outstretched fingers. 'Least said, soonest mended, ladies. I'll be back later.'

Checking the time on the ward clock, Kitty calculated that she had half an hour before she was due on the maternity ward. Casting an anguished glance back at her father, she wondered if her mother had received her telegram. Would she make it up to the hospital in the snow for a visit? Would Ned accompany her? How was her mother coping with the bitter-sweet news that her tormentor and the love of her life was desperately poorly? Had the police informed her that her incorrigible husband was back under arrest?

Trying and failing to silence the deafening din of her fraught thoughts, Kitty walked briskly to the ward where Dora Mackie was being looked after. At this hour, Sister Iris would be ensconced in her office, reading a book or else eating toast as the night shift neared its end.

Lily Schwartz was the first person whose eye she caught as she cracked the door open. Lily waved and approached when Kitty beckoned her over.

'Aren't you starting on maternity?' Lily asked, her voice barely above a whisper.

'I wanted to check on Dora. But I can do without a run-in with Iris.'

'Haven't you heard?' Lily said, grinning. 'She's "taking time off".' The mischief and delight in Lily's wide-eyed expression was obvious.

Kitty bit her lip. 'Do you think she's been suspended?'

Lily raised her eyebrows non-committally. 'The way she speaks to us all like we're dirt, it's the least she deserves. You reap what you sow. There's a different sister on. Henrietta. She's from the Royal Infirmary. Very nice.'

Feeling that it was safe to enter the ward, Kitty sought out Dora Mackie, who was awake now and sitting up in bed.

'Hello, love,' Dora said, immediately recognising Kitty. Her voice still sounded strange and tinny with the oxygen mask on, but it wasn't as sluggish as it had been before. She gestured towards the visitor's chair by her bed. 'I'm so sorry for what happened. I'm right ashamed. Especially after all you've done for me. How's your jaw?'

Kitty patted her hand. 'It's fine. Saves me putting on rouge.' She smiled and read Dora's notes, nodding enthusiastically. 'You seem to have turned a corner. Quickly, at that. Oh, that is good news.' She hooked the notes back on the end of the bed and patted Dora's hand. 'I'm so pleased. You'll be back home in no time.'

'They said I can try without the oxygen in a couple of days. Maybe even tomorrow.'

'What are you going to do about Mr Mackie? He won't be in the cells forever.'

'How do you mean?' Dora started to cough violently. When her chest settled, she couldn't look Kitty in the eye.

'If he punched me – a stranger – I don't need to be a genius to work out what happens to you behind closed doors. Dora, you've got to think of you and the children.'

Dora turned away. Her upper body started to shake.

'Don't cry!' Kitty said, standing up and laying a placatory hand on Dora's shoulder. 'Please. I didn't mean to upset you. I know how hard it must be. My dad's a handful.

It's always made life a misery for my mam. He was . . .'
How frank could she be with Dora? 'Let's just say he was
away during the war. I've never seen Mam so happy. She
thrived. Then he turned up on her doorstep and she's been
a doormat and miserable as hell ever since. And my dad was
never violent – just a sulk with a flair for cutting words.'

Dora looked back at her. 'He's fine most of the time.
I – I don't know if I've got it in me. I'm not sure I could
do it to him. See, he needs me and the kids.'

Kitty had seen it before on the wards – women who were
so lacking in self-belief that they couldn't envisage surviving
without being told what to do and where to go; the men's
love manifested in a hard slap at the end of a long night
spent in the pub.

'I'd like to get a holiday sorted for you and the children,'
Kitty said. 'A break somewhere lovely with fresh air. Get
them seen by the doctor, first, to do something about their
chests.'

'I told you we can't afford it.' Dora dabbed at her eyes
with the corner of her pristine white sheet. She winced as the
fabric skimmed over her bruising. 'The babies will be fine.'

'No, Dora. They won't. I'm praying they've not got TB,
but a doctor needs to examine them to be certain. In this
weather, you can't gamble with the lives of tiny, poorly tots.
We're living in a wonderful medical age, and our doctors
are prepared to waive—'

'Why are you interfering, when I asked you not to?' Dora
started to sob loudly, trying to pull her hands up to her eyes
but getting tangled in her drip. 'My Francis will go berserk.'

Digging her fingernails into the palms of her hands, Kitty
breathed in slowly. Castigatory words teased the tip of her
tongue, but Dora Mackie had been almost beaten to death.

Kitty wasn't about to shout at a woman who was already worn down to a husk. She exhaled and spoke quietly but clearly. 'It's *very* important that the children are treated, Dora. You're a caring mother, living in some tough conditions. I can see that. You're not a miracle-worker, though. You've got a lot of little'uns there, and it's freezing cold. Weather like this doesn't do babies any favours, and they *are* in a bad way. I know they've got a neighbour looking after them, but she's not their mam. It's not the same. Look, let's think about the children's safety. Let me help you, Dora. There are people connected to the hospital who can get you moved, maybe. Get you away.'

'My Francis loves me,' Dora snapped, clearly offended. 'I can never leave him. I took a vow in church before God. 'Til death do us part.' Her breathing was starting to sound ragged again.

Kitty realised she'd said as much as she possibly could – to no effect. She sighed inwardly and nodded. 'Sorry. Sorry. I didn't mean to – I understand.' What she really wanted to do was warn Dora that death had already paid her a visit and would be coming back with a sharpened scythe, if she didn't get away from her husband before he was released from the cells.

Chapter 33

Making her way to the maternity ward, Kitty groaned with frustration when she was certain she was alone on the corridor. She thumped the wall.

'Why?' she asked, looking at the ceiling as though God was floating above her head. 'Why is nothing ever straightforward?'

Her back felt bowed beneath the weight of her worries. Yet, she was about to start working on a ward where fresh life and new hope was brought into the dismal Mancunian darkness every day. That had to be worth something.

Come on, Kitty, she told herself. *Stiffen your spine and crack on.*

Within an hour, she'd been roped into assisting with a complicated breech birth in a side room, where the mother was no more than seventeen. As the exhausted girl laboured on her hands and knees, Kitty offered encouragement, holding her hand while the midwife tried to turn the baby.

'Don't push!' the midwife said. 'Not yet. Try not to push. Keep rocking back and forth.' Her tone was brusque.

Kitty noticed that the girl had no ring on her wedding finger. Was the midwife this abrupt with the married women who were admitted to the ward? she wondered.

'We're nearly there,' the midwife said, frowning as she gently tried to manoeuvre the upside-down foetus into the correct position. 'Doctor's coming any minute now.'

'Save my baby!' the girl said. 'Whatever happens, make sure he lives.'

The midwife tutted. 'You got yourself into this mess, young lady.' Then her tone seemed to soften. 'Don't worry. We'll get this babba out in one piece, come hell or high water. I've delivered thousands of little bundles and I've not lost one yet.'

Violet, who was standing by with a syringe full of pethidine, raised an eyebrow at the midwife's claim. Kitty wasn't about to delve deeper.

By the time the obstetrician arrived, delayed after having had to deal with a botched attempt at a home-Caesarean, the baby had been delivered. He'd been a slippery little package that had had to be teased out legs first, but when he'd emerged, it was clear he was a healthy boy with a good pair of lungs which were now shattering the peace of the ward. Kitty had stiffened with fear as the baby had been handed to her, enabling the midwife to deliver the placenta, but within moments, she was marvelling at his tiny balled fists and his purple-red face, scrunched up in a picture of pure fury.

'Jolly good,' the obstetrician said, taking the new delivery from her arms and examining him. 'You've got this all in hand, I see! Quite a first morning for you, nurse!' He swaddled the baby and set him gently in a tiny cot by the mother's bed.

The midwife looked concerned, however. 'Doctor, if you wouldn't mind taking a look at the mother.' She nodded pointedly towards the young girl, who was growing paler by the minute. 'She's torn badly. Losing a lot of blood.'

'Ah, yes. A little needlework for you, my dear,' the obstetrician told the mother. He turned to Kitty. 'How about you lend us some of your theatre expertise, nurse?'

Kitty assisted as the young mother was stitched up. Once the obstetrician was satisfied, she made her comfortable in bed. This was a world away from assisting in the normal operating theatre. Perhaps because two lives were involved, the stakes of any complicated admission seemed inordinately high. She was quietly considering how she might cope if she helped to deliver a stillborn, or if a baby died on the ward, when she heard a familiar voice behind her.

'Nurse Longthorne, do you have a moment?'

Turning around, she was surprised to see James standing in the doorway of the side room. At first, she beamed at him and blushed. There was no hint of a smile on his face, however. His demeanour was stiff and formal. There was no possibility of him bearing anything but bad news.

'Is it Dad?' she whispered.

He backed into the corridor, out of earshot of the new mother. 'I'm afraid it's not the best.' He looked up and down the corridor to check that they weren't being eavesdropped upon.

Kitty felt the blood drain from her cheeks. The ground beneath her seem to turn to rubber. 'He's not—'

'No. He's not dead. Far from it. He's woken up and is giving the policeman at his side rather an ear-bashing.'

Dare she allow herself a chuckle? No. 'So, no brain damage from the head injury? It's his spine, isn't it?'

James opened and closed his mouth, hesitating. 'I'm afraid he's got a nasty fracture of the spine. Lower vertebrae. He'll likely be paralysed from the waist down. At the moment, there's no feeling at all. I have a colleague at the Manchester Royal Infirmary, who studied under the famed neurologist, Professor Jefferson. He specialises in—'

'My dad's going to be in a wheelchair?' Kitty asked, blinking hard. She imagined the multiple flights of steep stone stairs that led up to her parents' flat in Salford Brow. How on earth would her mother and Ned cope?

'He'll be a paraplegic and wheelchair-bound at best. If his fractures heal. It looks that way. As I say, my colleague is going to take a look at him and see if anything can be done, but I'll be frank with you: he's lucky to be alive at all. You know as well as I do how high the fatality rates for spinal injuries are. Sepsis from bedsores and urinary tract infections always pose a tremendous risk in these circumstances. At the moment, your father's catheterised and being turned every hour. They're looking after his skin. The amputation site seems fine – for now.'

'Could your friend repair whatever's damaged? Dad's spinal cord, I mean.'

'Neurosurgery is a relatively young field, Kitty. I-I can't say for certain what his prognosis will be. I wish there was more I could do personally.' He looked down at his watch. 'I have to go. I have a meeting.'

'Don't you want me to fetch Violet? She's just dealing with a new admission.'

He reached out to take her hand and sighed heavily. 'No. Don't tell her I was here. Look, Kitty, there's been something I've been meaning to say since we were in the ambulance.'

Her heartbeat picked up to a steady gallop. James was looking deeply into her eyes. He opened his mouth to say something but paused.

'Go on! Tell me, for heaven's sake!'

Chapter 34

Whatever James had intended to say remained a mystery. Their impromptu tryst had been interrupted by one of his colleagues passing the maternity ward and drawing him into a discussion about a patient. Kitty had been left staring wistfully at James's back as he was ushered away – left in the dark as ever. She'd resolved to shelve her feelings and concentrate on her new role as a maternity nurse.

When her woefully delayed lunchtime swung around, despite her grumbling stomach, she opted to postpone a meal in favour of nipping up to see her father. It was already nearing the end of visiting time. Would her mother and Ned be by his side?

Fearing the condition he'd be in, Kitty entered the ward to find her father lying flat on his back with the bed tilted at some thirty degrees. His head sported a large dressing, rather than a bandage. Despite his bandaged arm stump and his spinal injury, he looked far more robust than he had on admission.

'Dad,' she said, nodding to the policeman and skirting round to the far side of the bed. She leaned over her father so that he could see her without moving his head.

'I can't feel my feet. In fact, I can't feel my backside, neither. But I can feel my arm, even though they've cut it off. They cut off my bleeding arm, Kitty!'

'You would have died if they hadn't, Dad. You were pinned under a flaming printing press the size of a bus.'

'And this toffee-nosed doctor come and explained stuff to me and I didn't have a clue what he was on about.' He managed to sound both belligerent and bewildered at once. He rolled his eyes towards the policeman. 'And this one's a barrel of laughs. He keep farting.'

'Dad! You've been in a very serious accident. What on earth were you doing underneath a printing press in a derelict bakery?'

'I'm saying nowt in front of *him*.' He clearly meant the policeman. 'I'll explain everything to the judge, if I must. This is a miscarriage of justice, this is. I'm a hero. I found an unexploded bomb that could have took half of Stretford out, didn't I? I literally gave my right arm to save lives, and they thank me by cuffing my left one to the bed.'

'You're not cuffed anymore. I think they've stopped worrying you're going to get up and walk off.' Kitty knew she ought to show her father more sympathy, but they'd parted under such strained circumstances and she knew exactly how heroic her father had been at the time of his fall. He could deny it all he liked, but the printing press and boxes of counterfeit coupons seemed fairly damning.

'It's a disgrace, is what it is!'

'Yes, Dad.'

'And the food is terrible. I couldn't get a meal 'til breakfast and it was rubbery porridge.'

'The hospital has to stick by rationing too, Dad.'

'Where's your mam? Where's our Ned?'

'I sent her a telegram. She'll be here. Maybe Ned'll drive her in the work van.'

As Kitty listened to her father moan about his lost arm and his crippling headache and the frustration and indignity of being 'manhandled' by young nurses on an hourly basis, she felt guilty at not being able to summon more sympathy. James was right. Most victims of spinal injury didn't make it. Their care was complicated and the risks were high. And yet, her father was a selfish man who blamed everyone else for his own shortcomings. He'd repeatedly told her the story of how he'd passed for grammar school but hadn't been allowed to go because his own parents, of course, could never have afforded the books and the uniform. Poor Bert Longthorne – a wasted intellect; he could have been a gentleman and a captain of industry, but for an accident of birth. Poor Bert Longthorne, who never forgot his duty to his family, though he was often gone for days on end and returned stinking of booze, cigarettes and women, with the pockets of his tailor-made overcoat stuffed with dirty money, which would later back a horse that conspired to lose. It was always a fix. In the meantime, little Kitty and Ned scraped by with whatever Elsie had been able to make from taking in sewing or charring for more fortunate women. The bile in Kitty's stomach bit at the sight of her father, excusing his misdeeds even after he'd been caught red-handed. The guilt that she should feel such anger and long-harboured resentment towards her own crippled father was far more corrosive, though.

'What's up with you, girl?' he asked. 'You've got a face like a cold fish supper.'

She was just about to give him a piece of her mind when she heard the doors to the ward open and a whimper from an instantly recognisable voice.

'Oh Bert! My Bertie! Look at you!'

It was her mother, and Kitty was relieved to see Ned following behind. Could this mean that he'd not been involved in the coupon swindle? She fervently hoped so. For once, she needed to believe in the menfolk in her family.

Greeting her mother with a bear hug, Kitty ushered her to the spare visitor's seat and eyed Ned with suspicion. It was hard to tell what he was thinking from his expressions alone. Severe burns and plastic surgery had afforded him the ultimate poker face.

'What a palaver!' her mother said, stroking her father's good hand. She started to weep. 'Oh, my Bertie. What in God's name have you been up to this time?'

Her father's eyes darted over to Ned. 'I was in the wrong place at the wrong time.' Then crocodile tears beaded at the corners of his eyes. Or perhaps they were genuine tears of self-pity. 'I can still feel my hand, even though it's gone. They say I probably won't walk again if an infection doesn't take me first.'

'Oh, they never!' Her mother was horrified.

Kitty had to intervene. She could see what was coming. 'Dad, they wouldn't have told you that. They don't know yet. Dr Williams is getting a neurology expert to look at you.'

'Dr Williams! Dr Williams! *That* pansy?' Her father grasped at her mother's hand. 'They're plotting against me, Elsie. I'm being fitted up. This is the hoi polloi ruling the working classes with a rod of iron. They're coming out with terrible lies about me. Once they've got their scapegoat, they'll finish me off. You'll see. Get me out of here, Elsie. Find the money for a proper solicitor.'

'Don't be daft, Bert. I had to throw the Welsh dresser on the fire this morning. Where in God's name am I going to find money for a fancy barrister?'

'I'm a cripple for life, love!' He looked at her with pleading eyes – all of his arrogance and aggression from the last time Kitty had seen him, before he'd stormed out of the flat, was gone now. There was calculation behind his eyes, however. What was he after?

No matter. Kitty left her parents to bemoan her father's condition and shoot accusatory glances at the blameless policeman. While they were preoccupied, she pulled Ned to one side.

'Are you involved in this?' she asked.

Ned shook his head. 'Of course not. I had no idea what Dad's been up to.'

She pointed to his disfigured face – a mess of scar tissue since the reconstructive surgery, though at least he had a nose, now. She knew he had several further operations on the horizon with James to finesse the crude miracles that had already been worked. 'All these surgeries. Where's the money coming from, now that the US air force isn't footing the bill?'

'Charity handouts.'

'Oh really?'

'Yes, really. Would I lie to you?'

'Well I wonder, *Dwight*!'

Ned looked at her shoulder. 'I'm a changed man, our Kitty. I know I had a lucky escape when I got involved with the wrong types before. I'm keeping my new nose clean with my job at the factory.'

'Well, I know that's not entirely true, Ned Longthorne,' Kitty said, narrowing her eyes at her duplicitous brother. 'Listen. Did you bring Mam here in your work's van?'

'Aye.'

'You got anything nice in the back? Any of that stuff you get from the GIs at Burtonwood?'

Ned shrugged. 'What for?'

'I've got a patient in serious need of a good cheering up. A lady.'

Ned scratched at his new nose and raised the eyebrow on the side of his face that had been left unscathed by fire. 'How about some perfume?'

Nodding, Kitty said. 'Like what? Nothing cheap. I don't want no rose water or Yardley. I'll pay, as long as I can afford it.'

'I thought you had nothing left, once you'd given Mam housekeeping.'

Straightening her apron, Kitty sniffed. 'I keep a bit by. And I expect a good price. You're my brother. Don't try fiddling me, Ned Longthorne. You're not too big for me to give you a wallop.'

Making their excuses, Ned led her to the place where he'd parked the van from the raincoat factory. He unlocked it and opened the back, showing Kitty some of the booty he'd acquired at Burtonwood to sell on to his neighbours in Salford Brow.

'Nylons?'

'No. Perfume. Like you said.'

Kitty ogled the brightly coloured packaging, noting Worth's *Je Reviens* and Guerlain among the boxes. She spied lesser scents, including *Tabu* by Dana, and soaps by Roger & Gallet. She picked up the Guerlain box that seemed impossibly chic. 'Is this the real McCoy? This is *Vol de Nuit*?'

'Fresh from Gay Paris.' He pronounced Paris as Paree, his teeth clacking in the icy cold wind that whipped around them.

Paris was a million miles away.

Kitty reasoned that a blast of something expensive and exotic might give Dora Mackie hope that life offered something better for her and her children. It might cost a struggling nurse a month's money, mind. 'How much do you want?' The will to do a good deed was far stronger than her need to set aside money for a rainy day. While she was a nurse, she was lucky enough to have her day-to-day needs provided for. Her mother had Ned to bring in a wage, these days. Dora was not so fortunate and though she'd probably appreciate the money more, Dora Mackie did not strike Kitty as the sort of woman who would take a handout. If she did succeed in giving her the money, Kitty was certain Francis Mackie would smell it from the far end of the street and burn it up at the tobacconists or drink it away in the pub.

Ned looked sideways at her, clutching his coat closed against the chill with one hand and weighing a box of *Je Reviens* in the other. 'Go on. You can have the Guerlain.'

'What!'

'I won a job lot of them at cards.'

It was more than cold that prickled its way up Kitty's back. 'Are you sure this isn't just bottles of tea with a posh label on it?'

'I swear.' Ned threw the perfume he'd been holding back onto the top of a wooden crate stuffed with fragrances. He took out a cigarette and sheltered inside the van until it was lit. He blew the smoke away from Kitty. 'You've got to stop worrying about me, our Kitty. I'm not the Ned that left for war.'

'Oh yeah? Is that why the back of your van's full of moody perfume?'

'French. Not moody.' He tried to grin, but the limitations of his scarred skin made it more of a grimace. 'Your patient will like that, anyhow. I hope she appreciates you. You're a thoughtful girl, our Kitty. Always have been.'

*

Taking her leave from Ned, Kitty smiled down at the bottle of Guerlain, feeling it would at least cheer Dora up. She made her way to the ward, realising her lunch hour was almost up. When she got there, the blood drained from her face and her fingers prickled. She dropped the perfume.

In place of the expected sight of Dora Mackie, lying there forlornly with a bandaged head, hooked up to her oxygen canister and chest drain, there was an empty bed. It had been stripped of its bedding.

'Oh my God! No!' she said. 'Don't tell me she's gone.'

Chapter 35

'Where's Dora Mackie?' Kitty asked the ward sister, fearing the worst. 'She hasn't passed away, has she?'

The sister looked bamboozled, momentarily. 'What do you mean, where is she?' She glanced at the empty bed and frowned. 'Who stripped that bed? That's odd. She hasn't been discharged. Not while I've been on duty. Doctor hasn't seen her since his rounds.'

'So, she's not dead?'

Striding to the empty bed and taking Dora's notes from the end of the bed, the sister scanned what had been written there. She shook her head. 'She's in absolutely no condition to have walked out. She's still mid-treatment.'

'Is there a note?' Kitty asked, still clutching the bottle of perfume that had mercifully not broken. She slid it into her pocket.

The sister shook out the sheets. 'No. Nothing. I can't understand why the bed's stripped.'

One of the trainee nurses was walking towards them, carrying a bedpan.

'Young lady,' the sister said. 'Do you have any idea what's happened to this patient?'

The trainee nurse blushed. 'She's been discharged, sister.'

'No she hasn't.'

'But she said she had been! Her husband packed her up and thanked us for looking after her.'

'Her husband?' Kitty said, feeling the spot where Francis Mackie had thumped her.

'Yes. Big feller. She left with him about half an hour ago – when you were dealing with a new admission. I thought I'd strip the bed, ready. You know? They're coming in thick and fast, aren't they, what with this weather and all? Did I do wrong, sister?'

Kitty left the hapless trainee nurse to bear the full force of the sister's wrath. How could Dora Mackie have walked out into the Arctic conditions with a punctured lung and terrible concussion? It was suicide!

Knowing that she had no opportunity to slip away from the hospital to check on Dora at home, given that her own family had to take precedence, Kitty returned to the maternity ward. There she found Violet, shaving a labouring mother in readiness for the delivery of twins.

'Lazy lunch?' Violet asked, rinsing the foamy razor in a bowl of water.

'I should be so lucky.' Kitty checked the clock on the wall. She still had one minute of her break remaining. Violet's implicit criticism stung and felt like the sort of comment that could easily sink its barbs into the hospital's grapevine. Kitty opted to distract her with a more personal nugget. 'My dad's been admitted.'

'So I've heard,' Violet said, pointedly. She exchanged a glance with one of the other nurses. 'You look positively harried, Kitty. I'm not surprised, given your family's *pressing* concerns.' She started to giggle. 'It must have been quite a *bombshell*.'

She'd heard about the printing press and the circumstances surrounding the discovery of the unexploded bomb.

That much was apparent. Kitty could see the mischief in her friend's eyes. 'How long did it take you to come up with those belters, Vi? Did you spend your lunch hour thinking up puns?'

'Me? Waste time on finding ways to poke fun at you, when I've got to *coupon* doing my best for these mums-to-be?' She laughed out loud at this juncture, apologising to her patient who glared up at her. 'Don't worry about us,' Violet told the labouring mother. 'We like to keep things bright and breezy on the maternity ward. It helps you ladies to relax.'

As Kitty resumed her duties by freshening up a labouring older woman, whose waters had broken far too long ago for comfort, she wondered if her new position on the maternity ward with Violet wasn't worse than what she'd endured on the nightshift with Sister Iris. How she wished she could work on the ward where her father was being treated, though she realised that would be a conflict of interest. It seemed that loathing him didn't preclude her from worrying about him.

Her morose imaginings of her father suffering from complications and having a sheet drawn over his grey, life-less face, were interrupted when Richard entered the ward. Their eyes locked immediately, and Kitty knew he'd come specifically to speak to her. She intuited by his grin that he wasn't about to deliver bad news.

When Violet moved closer, presumably to eavesdrop, Kitty felt like she was a strange exhibit in a gallery.

'Ah, there you are! My word, Kitty Longthorne. You're a difficult gal to track down. I've been looking for you everywhere!'

Kitty smoothed the edge of her nurse's cap with uncertain fingers. 'Matron transferred me. New ward; new shift.

What brings you here?' In her peripheral vision, she could see Violet who was pretending to fold cot blankets.

'I-I wondered if you might be free when you get off. We could see what's showing at the Curzon in Urmston, perhaps.'

Realising she ought to be flattered, Kitty forced a smile. 'Oh, Richard. That's sounds like a lovely – it's just that my father's very ill and I have to – I need to get over to check on my mother, too. There's a lot going on.'

Richard's cheeks coloured and his eyebrows shot up. 'Of course. Of course. Well, I could drive you. We can talk on the way. Where does your mother live?'

'Lower Broughton. Just past Strangeways. I told you when we went for—'

'Yes, yes. You did.' His expression said that if she had told him, he hadn't been listening. 'Well, I'm happy to take you in the Hillman, as long as you agree to accompany me for some supper on the way back.'

'Fine. Yes. That would be lovely.' Kitty could already hear the loaded comments that would almost certainly come her way from Violet, as soon as Richard left the ward. *Fancy accepting a lift off a single man! Going for supper, too! I bet I know what he thinks is on the menu!* But she was hardly going to turn down the opportunity to check that her mother was coping. The bus service into town was unpredictable at best in this weather, and then there was the matter of travelling another mile or two, out the other side.

'I'll swing by the nurses' home at eight?'

She nodded, watching Richard as he strode away with a visible spring in his step, whistling a merry tune.

'Ooh, you're a dark horse!' Violet said. 'Richard Collins, indeed. He's quite a dish! The second-most eligible man in Park Hospital. My word, our Kitty. Have you put a spell on him? He certainly seemed bewitched. Was it your earthy charm?'

'Who's the most eligible, then?'

'James, naturally! Though he's not exactly eligible anymore, is he?' She waved her glittering engagement ring in Kitty's face.

The hours trudged by with glacial slowness while Kitty clock-watched her way towards the end of the shift. Once the woman expecting twins had been safely delivered, the nurses had the opportunity to make a cup of tea – first, for the patients on the ward and then for themselves.

As they sat around Sister Gladys's desk with their drinks, Gladys turned to Kitty and looked at her expectantly. 'I see you had a visitor, earlier. Is this going to be a regular occurrence? Men visiting the ward for my nurses?'

Kitty scratched at the base of her neck. 'Dr Collins gave me a lift from town the other night. That's all. He knows I have to get from near Strangeways all the way back here, whenever I visit my family. He's just doing me a good turn.'

'A good turn involving a trip to the Curzon and a fish supper?' Violet asked, raising a shapely eyebrow.

'Take a powder, Vi! Really! I don't think sister needs to know my plans.'

The sister smiled knowingly at Violet and sipped her tea. 'Oh, there's no such thing as *just doing a good turn* when a fellow is smitten with a girl. I've had enough pretty young nurses like you on my wards over the years to recognise an infatuated young doctor when I see one.' She drummed her fingers on the table, oblivious to Kitty's discomfort. 'He's a handsome lad, though – and what a car! Tell me, is he an interesting sort? I've heard he likes blue films!' The hunger for gossip in the sister's eyes was clearly visible.

'He . . . err . . . I—' Kitty found herself flustered and unable to answer. She wasn't used to being the centre of attention.

'Did I tell you that James and I have finally set a date?' Violet blurted suddenly.

Like a dog, lured by a shiny ball, the sister's attention swung back to Violet, who took a dainty sip from a Royal Albert china cup that was painted with a 'V' on the bottom.

Violet smiled widely. Was it at the news she had just delivered or because she was now the centre of attention?

Kitty visualised James, standing at the front of a church festooned with summer flowers, awaiting Violet as she sauntered down the aisle in the Christian Dior gown she coveted. Her heart ached so acutely that she gasped. 'Let me guess. Will you be a June bride?' How could James do this, after he'd confessed his love for Kitty? Had they set the date before or after his revelation? Surely he'd have the time and the moral fortitude to back out of the arrangements if his heart didn't truly lie with Violet?

'Oh, no. We're not getting married in June! I've waited patiently enough. We're having an early spring wedding!'

'Next spring? Spring 1948?'

Violet trilled with laugher and patted Kitty's hand. 'Oh, you are funny, Kitty. No, this spring. We're getting married in four weeks' time.'

Had she heard correctly? Kitty held her breath and stared at the beaming Violet, desperate to hide the fact that she was crumbling inside. 'That sounds hasty. Had you set the date a while ago?'

'Last night. My mother's arranging everything. She's booking the most darling church in Bowdon. You should see the stained glass. Imagine the photographs! It's going to be a winter wonderland dream: a thousand white roses and acres of satin, trimmed with the finest white mink!'

'Last night?' Was it possible that James had sought out Violet after his confession to Kitty, wracked with guilt and all the more malleable for it? 'He's been fobbing you off for two years, but he decides to marry you inside four weeks – last night?'

'Whatever is the matter with that?' Violet said, wrinkling her nose and smiling quizzically. 'I love spontaneity. You can't beat it for being romantic.'

'It sounds terribly – shotgun, is all.' Kitty hadn't meant for her comment to sound like sour grapes but she was aware from the looks of horror on the sister's and Violet's face that she'd just said something incredibly uncharitable; bordering on catty.

'*Shotgun?*' Violet was flustered and blushing deep pink. She put a hand on her belly. 'I'm not sure I like what *that* implies. No, I think he'd just come to the conclusion that it was time. He's got to the place in his career that he'd set his sights on. He's a consultant on the board and an expert in his field. The only thing left to conquer now is me and fatherhood.' Violet took her hand off her stomach. Her grin was a show of teeth but the tightness around her eyes said she found Kitty's challenge disconcerting.

'I'm very happy for you both,' Kitty said. *Was* it feasible that Violet was pregnant?

As she set her cup back on her saucer, the tinkle masked the sound of her heart breaking.

Chapter 36

'Is this true?' Kitty asked, pulling James back by the sleeve of his jacket. The corridor was empty but for the two of them. Managing to catch him between surgeries and out of earshot of others had been tricky, but Kitty had always been on good terms with James's secretary – the keeper of his diary. 'About you and Violet marrying in four weeks' time – is she pregnant?'

He tried to detach himself from her grip as though she was a disgruntled patient on the offensive. '*Pregnant?* Good lord, no, Kitty! I have a meeting to attend.' He failed to look her in the eye. 'You're making me late.'

'You tell me you love me in the back of an ambulance but you still name the date with Violet? Really?'

He came to a standstill briefly, looking pointedly down at her hand on his arm. 'You're stepping out with Richard Collins, aren't you? He's been talking of nothing else in theatre. He's a good sort, you know, and you deserve happiness.' He gently lifted her fingers off the fabric of his jacket and patted her hand. 'You certainly deserve better than me.' She could see James was forcing an apologetic smile.

Kitty could feel the toast she'd hastily gobbled down in lieu of lunch, churning in her stomach. 'You're using Richard as an excuse. You're scared of Violet, aren't you? Or perhaps you just lied to me in the ambulance. It wouldn't be the first time you'd toyed with my feelings, James Williams. You never did tell me why you and me suddenly stopped being on the cards, and why Violet appeared in the frame instead.'

'It's complicated, Kitty. It's not just the promise I made to Violet, and how that would look if I reneged on it. It's my parents. Their expectations.'

It was no good. Kitty could feel white-hot rage fill her with incandescence that threatened to spill out through the palm of her hand in the form of a sharp slap. She had to get away from this ruinous bounder. 'Keeping up appearances, then? My God, James. You're so weak. And you're so cruel. Do me a favour, Casanova. Keep your feelings to yourself in future.'

Marching away from him up towards the ward where her father was being treated, Kitty kept her head down. She didn't want the oncoming gaggle of junior nurses to see her tears of frustration and disappointment. *No matter*, she thought, wiping her eyes. She would just keep going with quiet dignity as she always had in the face of adversity. *Violet's welcome to marry a man who doesn't truly love her.* Perhaps, that was the ultimate punishment for a pair of scoundrels who had lied and cheated their way up the aisle.

Was Kitty being too harsh? She shook her head in answer to her alter ego. No. Violet had never apologised. James had never explained. Both continually rode rough-shod over her feelings.

'I'm sick of it,' Kitty said under her breath. 'I've had enough.'

Half an hour spent by her father's bedside didn't improve her mood. He was still cantankerous but his condition had neither worsened nor improved. The young policeman by his bedside looked on the brink of despair, as he bore the brunt of Bert Longthorne's foul temper and sharp tongue.

*

Richard picked Kitty up at eight, sharp, and drove her through the spattering slush and flurry of virgin flakes into town.

'I think you'll love this film tonight,' he said, as the windscreen wipers hee-hawed back and forth against what was increasingly looking like a blizzard.

He started to explain which actors were on the bill and why the film he'd chosen to take her to had garnered critical plaudits in *The Times*, but Kitty wasn't listening.

'You know that I'm from a poor family, don't you, Richard?' she said, interrupting him mid-flow.

'I'd worked that out. Yes. And I know the circumstances under which your father was admitted. What of it?'

'Doesn't that bother you? Doesn't that – complicate matters?'

'Should it?' Richard looked over at her and grinned, looking almost predatory. He draped his arm across the back of her leather seat. 'Kitty, you're a lovely-looking gal, and I think your family background adds to your charm. You're so earthy and real. The working classes have a wonderful vibrancy that the middle classes don't.' His fingers seemed to be wandering awfully close to her breast.

Kitty shunted towards the door. 'I'd keep both hands on the steering wheel, if I were you. This weather's terribly treacherous.'

He removed his arm.

Kitty stared blankly out of the misty windscreen, considering his words. 'So, you find the working classes fascinating, do you?'

'Absolutely, I do. I love your camaraderie and drama. The folk music and food.'

'Folk music?'

'Irish jigs and that sort of thing. It's quite exotic to my Home Counties boy's eyes! The most excitement my parents ever had in Oxfordshire was the odd game of bridge or a visit from the vicar over tea and Victoria sponge. My mother's involved in the parish council. My father likes to play a spot of croquet on the lawn if his knees will let him. Nostalgic for the days when the summer air rang with the sound of leather on willow. He was a terrific batsman once upon a time. An Oxford Blue.'

'*Exotic?*' Kitty wanted to get out of the car there and then, but she realised she'd never make it safely there and back to Salford Brow if she relied on non-existent buses running late. Feeling Dora's bottle of Guerlain still in her coat pocket, she reasoned a cabbie would not accept that as payment either.

There was no need to spend the rest of the journey in awkward silence, given that Richard conversed for both of them, trotting out a monologue about post-war Britain being in a state of flux; the first time he'd knocked the family dog out with ether on a rag as an experiment; the glamour of Hollywood and how a National Health Service was both a blessing and a curse for doctors.

'How can it possibly be a curse?' Kitty asked as they rolled past Strangeways Prison – a monstrous, hulking silhouette of spires and jagged rooftops against the snow-laden night sky. 'People are still dying needlessly because they can't afford a doctor and are too proud to ask for charity. Half the nation can't see, for the want of an eye test and a pair of specs!'

'I'm just thinking aloud. None of us are in a rush to give up private practice entirely. I still make a respectable living from private surgeries in different hospitals. And I hope that won't change. The wealthy will always demand better, if better is on offer and can be paid for. It's just the way the world works, Kitty. If I were a barrister, say, why would I want to lie in an uncomfortable iron bed on a cold ward next to a coal miner?'

A barrister. Like James's father. Suddenly Kitty felt shabby in her second-hand boots and ungainly, outsized overcoat. She was relieved when the Hillman swerved its way up Derby Street towards the three- and four-storey blocks that comprised Salford Brow.

Approaching the building where her family lived, she spotted a man trying to lug a heavy-looking bag onto a wheelbarrow. It looked as though the barrow had tipped over in the snow, spilling its load. Kitty squinted into the darkness, punctured only by the odd shaft of yellow street-light. The fat snowflakes, lit like gold leaf in the sulphurous light, drifted down, settling on the man's shoulders in a cloak of celestial dandruff. He was familiar to her. As he turned to look at the approaching Hillman with undisguised suspicion, she realised why.

'Stop the car!' she said. 'That's our Ned!'

Richard pulled in slowly to the kerb and stepped out of the car, placing his trilby on his head and putting up his coat collar against the elements. He looked like an out-of-place gumshoe from a noir film.

'Ned!' Kitty scrambled over to her brother, embracing his freezing, sopping wet body.

'Aye, aye, our Kitty. How come you're over here? At this hour? Is summat the matter with Dad?'

'No, he's fine.'

'Well, what's with the toff in the getaway car?' He looked Richard up and down. 'Should I be running?'

'This is Dr Collins. He's given me a lift so I can check on you both. What *are* you doing?' Kitty asked.

'Coal. We're perished up there.'

'I say, old chap. Do you need a hand?'

Kitty could tell that Ned had already given Richard's impeccable overcoat a once-over by the sneaky grin that crept across his scarred face. 'You grab one end.'

Together the men hoisted the bag of fuel up the many flights of stairs. Both looked utterly dishevelled by the time they reached the top.

'Oh, what a lovely surprise!' Kitty's mother said as she opened the door. She caught sight of Richard and wiped her hands on her pinny. 'Come in. We're not proud.'

'Mam. I've been so worried about you since the episode with Dad.' Kitty clasped her mother close in a bear hug, wishing she could stay the night, here in the bosom of her family.

Before Ned closed the front door, Kitty noticed that he checked along the communal landing in both directions. He hung his damp coat over a clothes horse in front of the sorry-looking excuse for a fire.

'You expecting another visitor?' Kitty asked him, as he approached the window that faced onto the open-air landing and lifted the net curtain just enough to see out.

Ned shrugged. 'No. Just looking at the snow. You know? Wondering if it will ever stop.'

Kitty's mother seemed dumb-struck by Richard. She patted her hair beneath her scarf and smiled nervously.

'Let's get this fire going, eh?' Kitty said, slashing open the sack of almost certainly pilfered coal and filling the scuttle. She put six or seven blocks on top of the remaining glowing embers. Then she covered the aperture with a double sheet of newspaper so that the oxygen would be drawn down from the chimney, sending fresh, hungry flames upward.

They drank strong tea, served in old jam jars and sweetened with jam instead of sugar, which seemed to delight and entertain Richard no end. He regaled them with tales of Cambridge University and the fascinating history of anaesthesia, throwing in a gruesome anecdote of a soldier waking on the operating table, mid-surgery. They were so absorbed with his observations of how the other half lived that Kitty jumped when Ned, who had never entirely taken his good eye from the window, abruptly pulled on a coat and disappeared out of the front door. A flurry of paper cascaded through the air in his wake.

'Ned? Hey, Ned!' Kitty shouted after him as he ran pell-mell along the landing. He didn't turn back. 'What's got into him?' she asked, slamming the door shut and peering out of the widow. She just caught sight of him disappearing into the shadows of the stairwell.

Moments later, just as she and her mother had started to gather up the mess of paper, there was a thunderous knock on the door.

'Hang on, Mam,' Kitty said, her senses tingling. She felt sure from the aggressive thump, thump, thump, that this was neither her brother nor a social call. 'Let me.'

Before Richard could protest and take her place, Kitty had cracked open the door by only an inch or two. In her right hand, out of sight, she clutched the poker for the fire.

'Where is he?' The visitor was a man with stinking whisky breath and a deep scar that formed a sinister cleft down the side of his face. 'Where is that thieving little berk?' He pushed against the door and wedged his sodden shoe in the gap between the door and the frame.

'If you're talking about my dad, he's—'

'Not Bert. Ned. Who are you?'

'Who's asking?' Kitty kept her voice steady and pushed back so that the man's foot was painfully trapped.

He grimaced and put his face up against the crack. 'You tell him he owes me and I want paying. If he doesn't pay me by Friday tea, I'm going to take it out of his kneecaps. And if I can't get a grip of him, well maybe I'll take it out of you or your mam. I presume you're his posh sister.'

'Go to hell!' Kitty said, jabbing the poker through the miserly gap so that she hit the unwanted visitor in his soft belly.

He backed off just long enough for her to slam the door shut in his face.

'I say!' Richard said, standing decidedly further away from the door than Kitty's mother.

Kitty exchanged a glance with her mother. 'He's up to his old tricks, isn't he?' She took the stack of paper from her mother's work-worn hands and studied what was printed on it. 'Coupons? Counterfeit coupons. Crikey, Mam. Did you know?' Her hand started to shake as she realised the enormity of the discovery. She registered the sinking feeling in her stomach as a leaden mix of disappointment at her brother and fear for his safety.

Her mother shook her head vehemently. 'First I've seen of them. If our Ned had a stash of coupons, he was keeping them to himself. Look around you, Kitty, love. Do you see us living in the lap of luxury?'

'Has he had cash on him recently? Like, has he been unusually flush?'

'Oh, rot!' Richard said, fumbling through the coats that were hanging from the stand by the door. 'He's taken my coat.'

Kitty sighed. Of course he'd taken Richard's coat. She felt as though she was trapped in a gangster movie, where the projectionist's reel had become stuck, showing the same clip, over and over. Except this was no film noir, and Richard Collins was no Humphrey Bogart. 'I'm going to flipping murder him when I get my hands on him. Have you checked his bedroom recently, Mam?'

Her mother looked dumbstruck and shrugged. 'Why would I? He's a grown man.'

Kitty was just about to barge into Ned's bedroom to check for further evidence of misdeed when the window by the front door shattered and a brick landed with a thud by her feet. Attached to the brick by a piece of dirty string was a piece of soggy paper.

'There's a note!' Richard said, retrieving the brick.

Snatching it from him, Kitty stood amid shards of glass with an icy wind now blowing through the torn net curtain. She read the scrawled handwriting aloud:

'You're dead meat.'

Chapter 37

'You can't make any noise, Mam,' Kitty whispered, willing her mother to stop pottering and folding clothes and to come to bed.

'Nobody's going to—'

'Keep it down!'

Her mother dropped her voice to a whisper. 'Nobody's going to be listening out for me when you're working your shift. If they think you're on the ward, they'll not come looking for you here, will they?'

Kitty flung the eiderdown back, gesturing that her mother should abandon her tidying spree and get into bed. Finally, her mother relented and climbed into the narrow single bed, her head at the opposite end from Kitty's and her feet practically in Kitty's face.

'It was good of that Richard to drive us back. I was so embarrassed about our Ned taking his coat.'

'Don't lose sleep over his coat. We've got more on our plates than that. I had to endure an hour of Richard talking at me about Italian films. I reckon he owes me a coat!' Kitty made a mental note to pay Richard back somehow, in a way that wouldn't involve his hand up her skirt.

'Eh! I appreciate the risk you're taking, putting me up here,' her mother said.

'Just 'til that window's been fixed, Mam.' Kitty conjured a memory of the temporary repair she and Richard had bodged with some brown parcel paper and glue. The wind had still done its best to bite its way through four sturdy layers. 'Then you've got to report the brick to the police.'

'You know I can't do that.' The fear in her mother's wavering voice was audible.

'Well, unless Ned shows up with some money and pays that feller off, this problem isn't going to go away.' Kitty sighed heavily and stared at the streaks of light on the ceiling that came in through the chink in her curtains. It was so comforting to have her mother nearby – the warmth of another human in the bed reminded her of when she and Ned had slept top-to-toe as children, burrowing beneath the coats that had improvised as blankets. Her current circumstances couldn't have been worse, though.

She fell asleep trying to think of personal effects she might sell to pay off Ned's illicit debts. Except even her dog-tired, overtaxed mind was lucid enough to acknowledge that she didn't have a thing of value left in the world. And if, by some miracle, she did manage to clear his debts, she realised that he'd be in this exact same situation weeks, months or years down the road. It didn't matter how much time might elapse. The outcome would be the same. Ned was prone to bad decisions and getting involved with the worst kind of people. His father's criminally inclined blood ran thick through his veins. Kitty was certain that if Ned had fled to fight in the Far East, preferring his chances in a Japanese prisoner-of-war camp to his chances back in Manchester of dodging his debtors, he'd been involved in some dangerous and deeply unlawful behaviour before.

All night long, Kitty's dreams were awash with visions of the man with the fissure in the side of his face, peering in at her and trying to force his way into the flat. She was running through snow-bound streets that were dead ends; jerking herself almost awake when, in the dream, the scarred man had her cornered and swung a punch at her. He became Francis Mackie. Kitty transformed into Dora, trying to defend her babies. And each time, the nightmare ended with vivid red blood spattering across the white snow. It was a long, long night.

The following morning, the urge to get out of that cramped bedroom was intense. Kitty slipped her mother some bread and cheese and hastened over to the hospital to start her shift on the maternity ward. She arrived a good twenty minutes early, her head full of anxious ponderings as to how she could help Ned and convince her mother to move back to the south side of town.

The ward still had the night shift hush about it when she arrived. At first, she couldn't spot any staff at all – the only women she could see were mothers, walking up and down with their restless newborns or else lying in bed, breast-feeding.

Advancing down the ward, Kitty wondered if she was merely so tired that she was looking but not seeing.

'And that's not the half of it . . .' From behind a screen, Kitty could just hear Violet's voice. She was whispering and speaking quickly. 'You think it's a scandal that her father was caught red-handed with a bunch of counterfeiting hoodlums, trapped under a stolen printing press? Well, get this! Her father's been to prison.'

'A *jailbird*?' Violet's gasping co-conspirator sounded scandalised in the extreme.

Kitty drew closer, careful to make as little sound as possible. Though Violet might spot her feet on the other

NURSE KITTY'S SECRET WAR

side of the screen and clam up, Kitty was more than willing to be caught eavesdropping. She needed to hear the full extent of her one-time friend's betrayal.

'Yes. Three years in Strangeways for stealing balloon silk, I heard.'

'Wasn't she stepping out with your James at one point?'

There was the sound of shifting fabric. Was Violet wriggling uncomfortably in her seat? 'Well. That was a long time ago. We were quite close then, me and Kitty. I had my eye on James, but naturally, I wasn't going to tread on her toes.'

'No. Course not. Though they do say, "all's fair in love and war".'

Violet giggled quietly. 'I suppose I *might* have used my womanly wiles on James while Kitty was seeing him.'

'A love triangle!'

'It was only harmless flirtation, you know? He needed a little encouragement. *Doctor* James Williams and plain old Kitty Longthorne? That was never going to work, was it?'

'Did James know about Kitty's dad?'

'No. I don't think he did. But when I found out about her dirty secret, I soon disabused him of the notion that Kitty was anything of a catch.' She bleated high-pitched laughter, as though she was impressed by her own resourcefulness. 'She'd been lying to us all, after all. You can't trust a girl from a family of dead-legs like that.'

'Ooh, Violet. You are a one! But you're right.'

Kitty had heard enough. She reached out to whip the screen aside, revealing Violet in all her gossiping glory. Common sense stayed her hand, however, and she took a step back. If she confronted Violet, she'd be faced with the prospect of working on yet another ward with yet another enemy – there was no way that taking Violet to task wouldn't end in bad blood between them, and Kitty was sure she'd somehow end up in the wrong. Violet excelled at shrugging off blame. No, Kitty had been lucky to escape Sister Iris without incurring Matron's wrath. As it was, Iris had permanently transferred over to Crumpsall Hospital in north Manchester – out of sight and, finally, out of mind. Stoking a hornets' nest with Violet, however, would push Matron's patience too far. Instead, Kitty swallowed down the lump of hurt and padded noiselessly back to the entrance to the ward, where she made straight for the sister's desk and pretended to read the handover notes. On this occasion, it made sense to keep her counsel. Violet was a troublemaker, a heart-breaker and a liar, and as her workmate, Kitty was in the perfect position to keep an eye on chicanery.

'Morning, Kitty! How are you?' Violet asked when, finally, she emerged from behind the screen, closely followed by fellow nurse, Diane Godber – a notorious gossip.

Pretending that she had heard nothing of the slander, Kitty carried on as normal throughout her shift, though she was crumbling inside. Should she tell James that he had been manipulated? No. James should never have been susceptible to such scurrilous tittle-tattle, and Kitty was certain he'd taken Violet out on the evening of VE day, which had been hours *before* her father had climbed back into her life through the laundry window of the nurses' home. She now knew that she owed James nothing. He was a handsome rotter.

Matron, though, was a different kettle of fish. During her break, Kitty tracked her down on the ward where her father was being treated. It took several minutes to attract her attention as she pored over a file at the end of an elderly patient's bed.

'Have you come to check up on your wayward father, Longthorne?' She didn't take her eyes from the file initially. Then she smirked and looked Kitty in the eye. 'He's certainly giving Schwartz a run for her money. You'd think we were feeding him strychnine, not broth.'

'No. It's not about him. Can I have a word about something else, please?' Kitty's heart was beating loud enough to make her voice tremble and her hands shake. She looked over at her father who was indeed being fed from a bowl of soup by a flustered-looking Lily.

Narrowing her eyes, Matron cocked her head to one side. 'Oh? Is there a problem?'

'Not a problem, as such,' Kitty said. She pressed her lips together and held her breath momentarily. 'Just – It's Violet.'

Chapter 38

As the day wore on, Kitty wasn't sure if she'd done the right thing in telling Matron about Violet's slander. Much as she disagreed with her father's skewed moral code and the way in which he ran his affairs, she'd been brought up to believe one should never tell tales on people. On the impoverished streets of Hulme and Lower Broughton, a grass was a danger to the delicate balance of a community which relied on the cheap supply of stolen goods or employment opportunities that weren't exactly above board. Then again, she was a law-abiding citizen and was no longer prepared to be the butt of Violet's jokes.

Kitty looked over at her one-time-friend who was taking a blood sample from a woman who had been admitted with a suspected placenta praevia. Violet looked up. They locked eyes and Violet smiled sweetly as if she hadn't a care in the world. Had she been taken to task by Matron? Would Kitty feel a chill wind whipping through the ward when she had?

Without realising she'd been clenching her stomach muscles tight all day long, when her shift ended and she pulled on her cape, Kitty finally allowed herself to relax. She sighed long and hard, jumping when Violet burst into the storeroom where they kept their things.

'Hello, you! Any plans tonight?' Violet asked, taking a hand mirror out of her bag and pulsing her lips together until the flow of blood made them plumper and pinker.

Kitty looked at her blankly, imagining her mother slipping out from her clandestine hiding place in the nurses' home to find the makings of a sandwich. Perhaps she'd insist they make their way back to Salford Brow after dinner, to check on the flat and to see if there was news of Ned. 'Read a book. Do some knitting, maybe. I'm making a cardigan.'

'Quaint,' Violet said, her smile tightening. 'James and I are off to the church where we're getting married. There's *so* much to organise. We've allowed too little notice for a proper reading of the banns.' She blushed and clasped her hands to her chest. 'Imagine! All those years of engagement and, suddenly, we've got *four weeks* before we're Dr and Mrs James Williams!' She reached into her bag and pulled out a stiff cream envelope with a pink wax seal. 'Here. This is for you. We hope you can make it.'

With a trembling hand that she willed to be still, Kitty took the envelope from Violet. She fully realised what it contained. 'Thanks. I'll read it later when I've washed my hands and I'm sitting with a nice cup of tea.'

'Do open it now!' Violet's bright blue eyes glittered. 'I insist.'

'I've got to visit my father, Violet.' She slid the unopened wedding invitation into her own bag. 'Honestly, I'll savour it later when I'm less preoccupied with family worries.'

Violet stared at her, wide-eyed, perhaps not willing to believe that Kitty had said no to a bride-to-be. 'Of course. Of course. How is your father?'

Kitty swung her bag onto her shoulder. 'You mean, you don't know?'

'Why would I know?' Violet's smile froze on her lips.

Raising an eyebrow, Kitty shrugged. 'You seem to know a lot about my family. That's all.' She remembered Matron's words. *Leave it to me. You just get on with your work.* Now was not the time to start an argument with Violet.

Violet trilled with laughter. 'You talk about them all the time! I think everyone in the hospital knows the latest ups and downs of the Longthorne saga. It's like a radio play!'

'Well, I'm glad you're entertained. I'll see you tomorrow, Vi. Thanks for the invitation.' Kitty had to get away from her friend before she said something she'd regret. What James had confessed to her in the ambulance was so close to tripping off her tongue. The envelope in her bag felt heavy.

'Have fun with Richard!'

'I'm not seeing Richard.'

'Of course you are, you silly goose. He's *dishy*. And an anaesthetist. They're almost as good as proper doctors! Why wouldn't you see him?'

Putting one foot in front of the other, Kitty forced herself to walk away. 'Have a good evening, Violet. I really must go. Careful in the snow!'

In truth, Kitty had already decided that she had no real interest in Richard. She owed him a coat, after Ned's escapade, but she didn't owe him anything more. He was too self-absorbed; too flashy; too forward. She needed a humbler man; a kinder man.

Inadvertently, as she made her way along the draughty corridor, James crept into her thoughts – standing in front of a church altar, peering down the aisle at *her*, his handsome face lit up by his smiling eyes. She batted the ruinous imagining aside and entered the ward where her father was.

This evening, he was lying in bed, holding the *Manchester Evening News* up above him with his good arm, though Kitty knew he couldn't read and only ever looked at the pictures. The policeman at his bedside got to his feet and nodded at her.

'Miss.'

'Has this one been giving you any trouble?' she asked the constable. He was young and almost certainly fresh out of police college. His cheeks flushed when she spoke to him.

'Nothing I can't handle, miss.'

Turning to her father, she pushed the newspaper aside and kissed his forehead. 'Hello, Dad,' she said. He smelled of unwashed hair and medicinal alcohol. 'You look a little brighter than you did this morning.'

Her father threw the paper onto his nightstand. 'I've got a headache what won't shift and the dinner was lousy. My stump itches. Hey! That spine specialist from the Royal Infirmary came today. The one your feller knows.'

'Dr Williams? He's not my feller.'

'He had a good poke around. The spine doctor, I mean.'

'And?'

'He wants to operate. I told him I haven't got money for no operation, but he says he can get me in a wheelchair or maybe even walking again. With a stick, like. Says he'll do it for free.'

The door to the ward squeaked open and Kitty heard a man calling her name. She looked around, nonplussed. It was James. He strode towards her quickly.

'Here he comes!' her father said. 'Rhett Butler with a stethoscope.' He cackled mischievously.

'Ah, there you are, Nurse Longthorne,' James said. The furrows in his forehead were deep. His eyebrows knitted together into a dark smudge above sad eyes.

'Whatever's the matter?' Kitty asked, her heart thumping wildly beneath her nurse's uniform. Was it to do with Violet?

Was James about to castigate her for being confrontational with his fiancée? No. It was worse than that. She could see it in the tautness of his features, though to an outsider, he'd be a picture of professional composure.

'I-I need to speak to you. I have unfortunate news. It's come as a terrible blow. I'm so, so sorry.' He was toying with the fountain pen in the top pocket of his white coat.

She looked at her father and felt the blood drain from her own face, just as his paled. Had her father been mistaken about the promising prognosis from the spinal surgeon?

Turning back to James, she opened her mouth to speak, but he cut through her questions.

'She's been stabbed. She's dying.'

Chapter 39

'What do you mean, "She's been stabbed"?' Kitty said, leaping out of her seat with such urgency that the chair scraped against the floor and almost toppled backwards. 'Who's been stabbed? Who's dying?' She could hear the blind panic in her own voice as she pictured her mother being ambushed on a dark side street by Ned's debtors.

'Our patient with the collapsed lung.'

James was clearly being careful not to give a name in front of her father and the policeman, but Kitty knew he meant Dora Mackie. Her legs felt suddenly leaden and it was as though an invisible force was pushing down on her head and shoulders. Poor Dora. Tears – partly from relief that her own mother was safe but also deep sadness that Dora's life had taken another turn for the worse – bit at the backs of Kitty's eyes.

'She was admitted to casualty about half an hour ago with several stab wounds,' James said. 'She's in emergency surgery. I thought you'd want to know.'

Kitty turned to her father. 'I have to go, Dad. I'll be back in the morning.'

She didn't bother to kiss him.

Hastening down to casualty at James's side, Kitty thought briefly of how the Longthorne family life might have been, had her own father been a wife-beater, rather than a morose and selfish sulk with bad judgement and worse friends.

Please don't die, Dora. Please hang on in there! she thought.

269

'I don't know why this particular patient has affected me like this, after all these years,' James said, as they headed down the corridor towards the tiled glare of the operating theatre. 'Losing patients is part of being a doctor.'

'And of being a nurse,' Kitty said, remembering the horrors she'd seen during the war. She sighed. 'I think we just got involved this time. Both of us.'

James took her hand and slowed her down.

'What are you doing?' Kitty looked down at his hand and shook him off. 'Enough of—'

'I've got agreement and funding for a trip to the Alps. Just this morning, in my meeting. For Dora and her children – and others like them, suffering from chronic respiratory problems. Baird-Murray knows this philanthropist. A few of us were also going to chip in.'

Kitty could feel her spirits falling like mercury in a thermometer on the coldest, darkest day of the year. She swallowed hard. There was no time to respond, however. The doors to the theatre loomed before them.

'Who's operating?' Kitty asked.

'MacBride,' James said. 'He's a good surgeon. But I think one of the wounds had punctured her liver and there's internal bleeding.'

Pushing open the doors, they both donned surgical attire and scrubbed their arms to their elbows. When they were ready, Kitty led the way to the operating table, but hung back to allow the surgeon and surgical nurses to work on Dora. Everyone working to save Dora's life worked calmly and efficiently, but it was a bloody scene with grim resignation hanging in the air.

'Come on, Dora,' Kitty said, though Dora was deeply asleep with a drainage tube in her mouth. 'Stay with us.'

Might Dora hear Kitty?

'You and the kiddies can go on a lovely holiday after this,' she said, wishing her words of encouragement weren't so pointless.

Dora wasn't listening, however. Dora wouldn't hear a comforting voice ever again.

'She's gone,' MacBride said, taking a step back and holding his bloodstained hands aloft, almost as a gesture of defeat. He looked at the clock and spoke solemnly to the nurses. 'We've done everything we can, ladies. Time of death is twenty to nine in the evening.'

'Oh!' Kitty felt as though she'd been thumped in the throat, and tears fell regardless of whether they were appropriate for an experienced nurse or not.

Dora Mackie's punctured body looked so lonely on the operating table. Kitty gingerly stepped forwards and held her hand.

'Goodbye, Dora,' she sobbed. 'I'm so sorry to see you go. I'm so sorry for all that's happened to you. I wish you peace.' She tried to hold the tears back, but they trickled over her cheeks – one onto her top lip, the other onto her jaw, skirting the tender place where the bruise left by Francis Mackie still lingered.

James put his hand on her shoulder and led her away from the glare of the theatre's lights, away from the judgemental eyes of the surgical staff. 'I wish we'd done more.'

She leaned into him and rested her head on his chest, beneath which she could hear the steady, reassuring beat of his heart. Then she allowed herself to weep until the sadness and anger rolled back like a receding tide.

'I hope the police get him,' she said. 'I hope they lock that murderous bastard up and throw away the key.'

'They will,' James said, kissing the top of her head.

Kitty pulled away and met his troubled gaze. 'What will they do with her children?'

He shook his head. 'Perhaps she has a surviving female relative.'

'She mentioned an aunt in Rawtenstall.'

'I'll make enquiries. I promise. I'll make sure they're seen by a doctor. Maybe Galbraith will have them in his clinic, if they're sick enough to warrant it. Francis Mackie should hang for this.'

Kitty returned to her room to find her mother was sitting by the fire, stirring an old cooking pot of something that smelled delicious.

'Where's all this food come from?' She took the wooden spoon from her mother and stirred thick brown goo with white lumps in it.

'It's stew,' her mother said. 'Fish stew. I nipped back to Salford Brow. We had food what wanted using in the scullery. Parsnips and spuds and that. The fish is summat called snoek. From South Africa. I had a couple of tins in and got this recipe from Irene, two doors down, called *Snoek Piquant*. Not that I had any of the other things to go into it!'

'It looks –' Kitty wrinkled her nose at the strange fishy lumps in gravy. 'You shouldn't be cooking in the room, mam. You can smell it right down the corridor. People will get suspicious.'

'Cobblers to that! I was hardly going to waste it, was I? Not when I've got no more coupons 'til next week. Not legal ones, anyhow.'

'Crikey, mam! I could have smuggled you out something from the dining room. Why did you go back to Salford

Brow? It's dangerous!' Kitty said, shedding her coat.

'I checked the coast was clear. I was in and out. Didn't speak to no one.' Her mother looked sheepishly down at her hands. 'The place had been turned over.' She laughed mirthlessly. 'Good job we've got nowt worth nicking. I straightened everything back up and went to the rent office about getting the door fixed and the broken window. There was frost on the *inside* of the walls, can you believe it? Talk about brass monkeys. Anyhow, they sent someone round. I've been busy. But I didn't want to stay there. Not with our Ned gone to ground and some hoodlum knocking around.'

Kitty swallowed hard. 'Oh, I'm so glad you're here with me, Mam,' she said, embracing her mother tightly and squeezing her eyes shut lest she imagined Dora Mackie's lifeless body on her own bed. 'Thanks heavens you're safe. We'll get you a new place. I promise.'

'What about my boy though? I feel like I've only just got him back. Oh, Kitty, do you think he'll be all right?'

'Our Ned? Listen! He managed to escape the Japanese and travelled across the whole of Asia on foot! I'm sure he can look after himself in the wilds of Salford. Don't lose any sleep over him.' Kitty kept her own worries about her wayward brother to herself. 'Our Ned will show up like a bad penny. He always does.' Her voice started to wobble and suddenly, Kitty felt a wave of sadness overwhelm her.

Her mother pulled off her nurse's cap and stroked her flattened hair. 'Hey! Hey! Shush. Shush. Shush. Come on! Tell your old mam. What's up? Have you had a bad day, love?'

Kitty nodded. 'I lost a patient. Oh, it was so sad, Mam.' She pulled a cotton handkerchief from her skirt pocket and dabbed at the tears. Then she held her mother's hands and stared into her bloodshot eyes, noticing the red split veins on her wind-burned cheeks and the laughter lines around a mouth that was beginning to prune ever so slightly. 'She reminded me of you.'

'Oh, ta very much!' her mother said, raising a sceptical eyebrow.

'She had a bad husband, I mean. Worse than Dad, but – I don't want to see you end up in hospital because of Dad or Ned. You deserve better, Mam.'

Kitty's mother pressed her lips together and exhaled heavily through her red-tipped nose. Her breath steamed on the cold air. 'You're right. I do. I never wanted to be married to a sulking jailbird what can't keep his fingers out of the till. When I met your dad, he was a handsome young man, doing an apprenticeship as a joiner.' She stared wistfully at the cooking pot. 'He turned up at your gran's for our first date, dressed to the nines with a posy of beautiful flowers. Said he was going to take me to the Midland for afternoon tea and then to the Gaiety Theatre over the road for a show. There's me in my Sunday finery, hoping to be treated liked a lady. Turned out, he had nothing planned at all.' She chuckled. 'And the flowers he'd nicked from a grave! We ended up sitting in Alexandra Park on a bench with a bag of scrapings from the chippy, watching a brass band on the band stand! I should have known what he'd turn out like.' She kissed Kitty's head. 'But at least I've got you to show for it. You and Ned. You're everything I could have hoped for in a daughter. I'm so proud of you, our Kitty! And I still believe your brother can mend his ways.'

'He's got a good heart.'

'And if your dad survives, he'll need me to nurse him. How can I turn my back on the big lump in his hour of need?'

Kitty sat up straight and stiffened. 'If Dad survives, he's going back to prison.'

'Don't kid yourself, Kitty, love,' her mother said, rising to stir the stew. 'Your dad will do anything to avoid another spell in the clink. If there's a chance he can get off with a rap to the knuckles in return for blowing the whistle on the others, he'll take it. He whispered it to me when I first visited him in hospital. He said he'd take care of everything and he winked.'

'Dad's going to grass? Never!' Kitty thought about a childhood being preached to about the importance of loyalty and of never running with tales about others – a corner-stone of sometimes questionable Longthorne morality. She considered how conflicted she'd felt about ratting Violet out to Matron.

'Your dad's always looked after number one.'

Kitty curled her lip. 'What a hypocrite!'

As Kitty ate her stew, listening to her mother's hopes and fears about finding a new home within travelling distance of her job at the raincoat factory, she wondered how it was that men made the rules that bound women but seemingly never thought twice about flouting them themselves. She thought about Francis Mackie, stabbing his devoted wife to death. She thought about her own father, who bungled and burgled his way through life with no thought for the penal – or the moral – code. She thought about James, the lying doctor, who had promised his heart to a socialite's daughter but who was clearly still in love with a lowly girl from Hulme.

In the middle of the sleepless night, Kitty donned her overcoat and left her mother snoring gently. She trudged back over to the hospital, braving the hard crust of ice that covered the inadequately gritted path. Looking up at the window to James's office, she saw there was a light on.

'Ha! I was right,' she murmured to herself.

He was a man who slept little and worked too much, Kitty knew, as if his clinical caseload would save him from the difficult business of conducting human relationships.

Squinting in the harsh light of the empty, draughty corridors, she ventured upstairs and knocked on the door, her heartbeat thundering away.

'Enter!' he said.

She found him sitting at his desk, making notes in a file – suited and immaculately groomed, as though it were ten in the morning rather than three.

'Kitty!' He looked perplexed at first, then smiled warmly. He stood up and gestured that she should sit down. 'To what do I owe the pleasure of a night-time call? You're not on the night shift, are you? Surely you should be tucked up in bed. It's the witching hour!'

Remaining standing, Kitty folded her arms tightly across her chest. She knew she looked absurd in the knitted hat and many layers of clothing, but she didn't care. She had to stop living life by silly rules and double standards. She had to get this off her chest. She forced herself to blurt the words out.

'I love you, James Williams, and you love me too, you idiot man. Are you really going to marry Violet, when me and you could be together?'

James looked at her, clearly dumbstruck. The smile hardened on his lips.

Chapter 40

'What's that you've got there?' Kitty's mother asked, trying to read the stiff card that she was holding before her.

'Nothing,' Kitty said, hastily shoving the invitation back inside her bag. 'Just an order of service for the funeral.'

Some two weeks had passed since Dora's death. Kitty was sitting on a settee that had been salvaged from the rag-and-bone man's handcart in her mother's new place – a 1930s ground-floor maisonette in Ordsall which had been earmarked for demolition, once Clement Attlee's new government had finally decided what to do with Manchester's and Salford's bomb-pitted slums.

'Oh, right. Make sure you keep well wrapped up, then. It's cold enough at the cemetery as it is, let alone with ten-foot snow drifts.'

'I've got my thermals on, Mam.'

'Hey! Did you hear? There was a trawler what sunk just outside Grimsby the other day, because of the gales and ice and that. It's never ending. I like snow as much as the next woman, but after weeks of burning whatever I can get my hands on to keep warm, I'm sick of the stuff.'

Kitty kept her pain at the thought of James marrying Violet in only two weeks' time to herself. She offered her mother a hearty smile. 'Count your blessings, Mam. If the old lady who had this place before you hadn't frozen stiff in that armchair –' she pointed to the winged armchair that

277

had been left behind by the previous occupant – 'you'd still be sleeping top-to-toe in my bed in the nurses' home, having to pay rent on a flat you weren't even living in.'

'Aye, well, I'm glad to be out of Salford Brow. It's a bit rough near the Barbary Coast—'

'For heaven's sake, Mam. Keep away from the sailors. Those docks bring nothing but trouble and debauchery.'

Her mother gave her a dismissive wave. 'This place'll do me for the time being. I'm thankful to have a roof over my head at all after that nonsense with the coupon swindle. I was lucky the police believed I knew nowt about it.'

'You're lucky Dad's cut a deal with the coppers, you mean. And Ned's done you a favour by hoofing it to Liverpool.'

Her mother ignored the barbed comments. 'When he comes home, your dad can sleep in the front parlour.'

Much had happened in the last fortnight. After using her free evenings to trawl the pubs of Lower Broughton, Salford and Trafford where Ned and his associates were regulars, Kitty eventually discovered that Ned had absconded to Liverpool and was 'dossing' in the attic of an old friend from his battalion in Bootle. Getting around in the snow had been an arduous task. On more than one occasion, Kitty had hitched a ride into town on a horse-drawn sledge, since many drivers had been unable to fuel their vehicles in the abnormally cold snap, due to blocked ports.

Finding the maisonette had been relatively easy through a network of well-meaning washerwomen who serviced the hospital's laundry. Kitty had helped her mother to move house with nothing more than a handcart. Though James had offered to load his car with her meagre belongings, Kitty had turned him down, preferring to struggle the three and a half miles in the snow, on foot, than to accept his insincere charity.

There lay the rub. For all James had made the spinal surgery possible that looked as though it might restore some of her father's mobility and would certainly save his life; for all James had stood in his office two weeks earlier at three in the morning and had confessed that his heart would only ever belong to Kitty; for all they had kissed passionately, – a kiss that had electrified her in a way she'd never thought possible, so that even when their fingertips had touched, she'd felt a jolt of energy that could have lit up the whole hospital in a power cut – he was still marrying Violet.

'My father will disinherit me unless I marry her,' he'd said, having broken the passionate spell with the painful truth. 'It was Violet that told my parents about your background, long before your father was let out of prison. I'm so sorry. It was complete coincidence. You and I had started courting, but Violet and her mother had met my mother at a ladies' bridge party at the Jones's house. I didn't realise until recently why my father had been so insistent that I break things off with you and step out with Vi instead. But he was adamant, Kitty. If I continued to see you, he'd cut me off entirely.'

'Does money mean so much to you, James Williams?' Kitty had said, feeling like the wind had been knocked from her with a hefty punch to the gut. 'Could you not have stood up to him? A man in his thirties, cowed by his own father?'

'I don't give a fig about my inheritance. But my father is a major contributor to a charity that I founded.'

'I don't believe you! What charity?'

'The Face the Day Foundation. It's for people with facial disfigurements. Much of the money funds the unpaid reconstructive work I do on ex-servicemen and burns victims. Like your brother. Research into new techniques, too. Unless I marry Violet, my father has threatened to withdraw his financial support entirely. How can I say no to the funding that changes so many people's lives? And how could I condemn you to married life with such a hateful snob as your father-in-law? You're too good for that, Kitty!'

Kitty had been faced with the brutal reality of James's situation. To be with him, she'd be stealing hope and a future from men and women who had had everything else stolen from them by the war. To let him go, she'd be abandoning him to a loveless life with the vain and shallow Violet: every bad boy's dream; every good man's nightmare.

They had parted company in the dead of night – she, in tears, he, ashen faced. Kitty had had to resolve to support James in his decision for the good of his patients. She had never felt so wretched as she had on that long, cold walk back to the nurses' home, knowing she had willingly given up the fight for the love of her life.

The only positive things that had come from the tragedies of the last two weeks had been Kitty's father's seemingly successful surgery (though only time would tell to what extent he'd regain his ability to walk) and his apparent evasion of arrest for the coupon debacle. There was also the conviction of Francis Mackie. The small clipping in the *Manchester Evening News* had told her that he'd been sentenced to death by hanging, with the date still to be set. The Mackie surviving children had *gone to live with relatives*, according to the reporter, but not until their chest infections had been treated by the cardiothoracic specialist, Mr Galbraith.

Outside, there was the rumble of a car's engine and a squeak of brakes. Kitty saw the black bulk of the Ford Anglia through her mother's dingy net curtains.

'I've got to go, Mam.'

She pulled on her black gloves, hat and coat, kissed her mother goodbye and headed out to meet her companion on this most unhappy of mornings off.

The neighbours' curtains were twitching as her driver for the occasion got out of the idling car and opened the passenger door for her.

'Ready?' James asked. His face looked pinched in the sub-zero temperatures; his breath billowed like a dragon's, mingling with the car's exhaust fumes and the freezing mist that rolled in from the nearby docks. In his Saville Row-tailored funeral attire, he looked more like a Hollywood silver screen star than ever.

'Let's pay our respects.' Kitty put her hand on his shoulder momentarily, brushed an imaginary speck of dust away and folded herself into the car in as ladylike a fashion as the weather conditions allowed. 'Does Violet know where you are and who you're with?'

He shook his head and closed the passenger door.

Kitty felt another pang of regret and disbelief as he made his way around the bonnet back to the driver's side. He climbed into the Ford, bringing with him a smell of expensive aftershave and a suggestion of how her life might have been, had Violet not flung such an impassable obstacle in the path of their true love.

'Do you think they think I'm a gangster?' James said, gazing at the gawping neighbours.

Kitty smiled wryly. 'Round here? I reckon they're thinking you're my pimp.'

The funeral was a sorry affair in the freezing cold St Ann's Catholic Church in Stretford. As Dora's simple coffin was carried in, led by the priest and borne on the shoulders of diminutive men who were almost certainly no blood relations of the behemoth, Francis Mackie, Kitty wondered that the murdered woman could have been so tiny.

'It's like a doll's coffin,' she whispered to James, only just audible above the church's organ that played a mournful hymn.

'She was very underfed,' he said. 'If this rationing continues for much longer – especially with the blight that's affecting crops in this weather – people will be starving to death in droves.'

Only the oldest child was present, sitting with an elderly woman, whom Kitty assumed was Dora's aunt. Dressed in a black suit that was too big for him, with flame-red cheeks from the cold, the boy cried quietly throughout the Mass.

'Are you a religious woman, Kitty?' James asked, as the congregation took their turn to receive Holy Communion.

Kitty turned to him and frowned. 'I wasn't even baptised, me, but my gran on Dad's side was a lapsed Catholic. My granddad was Church of England. Mam's parents – I've no idea. God didn't seem relevant in our house. I don't think I've thought about him in a long, long time. If Jesus *is* up there, looking down on us, well, he can't be looking very hard if he lets women like Dora be murdered in their beds. And he seems to have turned a blind eye to the slaughter of millions of soldiers and civilians in the war and all.' She sniffed hard and looked at the dazzling golden statuary on the altar, then lowered her gaze to take in the sorry sight of Dora's coffin, festooned with a simple Holy Bible. There were no flowers – unsurprising, given the cold snap. 'Or maybe that's just the fallibility of man for you. What about you?'

James sighed. 'My family's Anglican, but I only believe in the salvation offered by medicine, I'm afraid. I don't think you need the Church to know right from wrong. Violet disagrees. She thinks a nice church makes a terrific backdrop to a wedding portrait.'

Kitty was certain he rolled his eyes, though his obvious disdain for his own fiancée wasn't enough to alleviate her own crippling hurt. Violet was still the woman who would get to spend the rest of her life by James's side. Violet would share his bed and bear his children. What did Kitty have beyond her modest career? A spinster's future, clucking over her put-upon mother and ailing father; worrying about her wayward brother, who would be heading either for prison or the cemetery, if he didn't mend his ways.

Thankfully, her attention was drawn to the priest, bent almost double and clearly in poor shape, who mounted the pulpit with almost glacial slowness.

He read from the Gospel and started to deliver a homily, reflecting on the passage he'd read. It was followed by a stultifying eulogy about a woman he hardly seemed to have known at all, though Dora had told Kitty she'd been a regular churchgoer. Towards the end of the speech, the priest spoke with more passion. He seemed to grow in stature and leaned on his lectern to stare at the congregation.

'Why did the Lord choose to take Dora, a mother of five, in this bitter winter of discontent?' he shouted in a Cork accent that seemed to roll its way along the Stations of the Cross until every corner of the church rang with it. 'Here was a woman who served God and she *shall* join Him in heaven. But the country her husband fought for and the government she paid her taxes to failed her!'

Kitty looked askance at James. He raised an eyebrow in response.

'She was left to go cold. Her children were left to go hungry. Her husband was left to go mad with the horrors of war. Here was a poor working family that gave everything to Queen and country but got nothing in return. Where was the earthly reward for Dora? Where are the homes we're promised? Where is the food for our table? Where are the doctors to cure the sick?'

At her side, James's Adam's apple rose and fell. He looked down at his knees, his brow furrowed.

Kitty squeezed his hand. 'He's got more front than Woolworth's, that one! The Church has always got its hand out. Listen, we know we did right. Take no notice,' she whispered.

The priest's sermon swung back towards more spiritual matters and a more palatable notion of Jesus feeding the hungry, perhaps where rationing failed. No matter. His words had had a profound effect on Kitty, and she was more desperate than ever for the introduction of a National Health Service that would stop so many tragedies before they began. She knew James would be feeling the same.

Afterwards, once the coffin had been incensed and sprinkled with holy water by the priest, then loaded back onto the horse-drawn hearse for the committal, she followed James to speak to Dora's aunt.

James extended his hand to the older woman, whose eyes were the ragged red of the bereaved. 'I'm so sorry for your loss. Mrs Ferry, isn't it?'

She nodded, holding Dora's oldest son close. 'Who are you?'

'I'm the doctor from Park Hospital who operated on her when she – fell down the stairs. Dr James Williams.' He gestured to Kitty. 'This is Kitty Longthorne, the nurse who saved your niece's life that time, by whisking her to theatre.' He looked at Kitty with eyes that seemed to glitter, though it could have been a reflection of the frosty glare from outside. 'Kitty went to your niece's house to check on the children. We've both been following Dora's plight.'

The aunt's face was crumpled with bitterness. 'Aye, well, you didn't do nowt, did you? She still ended up with a knife in her belly.'

James nodded. 'It's terribly tragic. But we want you to know that we're going to be in touch about a trip for the children. To the Alps.'

The aunt treated him to a withering sneer. 'You what?'

'Fresh air and mountains. It will be restorative.'

'Mountains, my arse. They'll catch their death up there.'

'On the contrary, Mrs Ferry. If things persist as they are, they'll catch their death down here.'

Kitty could see by the aunt's sharpening eyes and hard, pruning mouth that they were on the brink of an ill-timed argument. She laid her hand on James's arm. 'Not now. Come on.'

She led him away. They drove back to Park Hospital in silence.

It was the last time they spoke until the day of James's and Violet's wedding.

Chapter 41

'Typical,' Kitty said, peering out of her window at the spring sunshine. 'If she fell off a mountain, she'd fall into a divi-ticket at the Co-op, that one.'

The last heavy snows had fallen on 15 March and the melt had begun, just in time to allow Violet a chilly but bright spring day for her marriage to James at an idyllic-looking old church in Bowdon. Her socialite mother had invited everyone who was anyone and a hundred more besides, if Violet was to be believed – theatrical types, chanteuses, at least two politicians, artists, famous novelists and the great and the good of the medical world. Every day, she regaled all on the maternity ward who would listen with each and every detail of the big day's planning.

It had pained Kitty to listen, but she had smiled politely, hopeful that her crushed spirits would go unnoticed if she squashed into a pew near the back. If Matron had had words with Violet over her gossip-mongering, Violet hadn't shown it.

Now, standing in front of her mirror in her Spartan but impeccably tidy room, Kitty pulled her new floral dress over her panty girdle and well-upholstered bra. She sighed heavily and tugged at the heavy fabric which she was certain had been cut from a stolen bolt of curtaining chintz.

'Matronly. That's what you look,' she told her reflection. 'No. Forget matronly. You look like a flaming armchair. Veronica Lake, eat your heart out.'

Kitty had paid for the dress to be made by one of the seamstresses at the raincoat factory where her mother worked. Her old dress 'for best' had been made when she'd been only twenty. Fashions had moved on in those years and though still trim, with a small waist, Kitty now had filled out to cut a more womanly, hourglass figure. Still, she realised that this new dress, though the sleeves were the correct length and the top accommodated her larger bust, was hardly *en vogue*. When Violet sashayed down the aisle in her Christian Dior-inspired 'new look' wedding gown, Kitty would feel exactly what she was. An interloper. An unwanted guest. A shabby offcut. Knowing that the groom didn't love the bride and hankered after Kitty instead was no consolation whatsoever.

'Why am I doing this?' she asked herself, licking her eyeliner brush and dabbing the tip into the soot at the back of the fire grate. She carefully drew lines on her upper lids and blackened her lashes. Finally, she applied some Max Factor blood-red lipstick that Ned had got her from lord-knew-where, but which was starting to smell decidedly stale.

The transformed Kitty stared back at her. She decided she looked like a harlot in a loose settee cover, but there was no time to change either the dress or the make-up. A charabanc was waiting outside to take a large gathering of nursing staff and those doctors who lived nearby to the church.

'Oh, heck. I'll have to do.'

Kitty pulled on a hat and smart red coat she'd borrowed from her mother's new neighbour, who was by far the most elegant (and only) brothel-keeper she'd ever met. Finally, she slipped on freshly polished shoes that had seen far too little dancing and snatched up the carefully wrapped wedding gift of a fruit bowl. As she made her way downstairs and out to the other excited guests, she idly sang the old song her mother had sung whenever she'd red-raddled the step of their old house – *Why am I always the bridesmaid, never the blushing bride?*

'You're an idiot, Kitty Longthorne,' she told herself as she waved to Lily Schwartz.

Just as she was about to mount the steps of the charabanc, a car tooted its horn merrily and Richard Collins pulled up beside her in his shining Hillman.

'You're a sight for sore eyes, Kitty,' he said, grinning at her as though she'd never turned him down. She could see that he was all dressed up in tie and tails for the wedding. He gestured to the passenger seat beside him. 'Hop in and we can arrive in style.'

Kitty looked longingly at the car, imagining the Hillman sweeping up outside the church in a part of Cheshire where the air was so rarefied, Kitty had only ever read about it in dog-eared copies of *The Tatler & Bystander*, borrowed from Violet. The periodical frequently covered the coming out of new debutantes at Bowdon and Dunham balls, where the champagne flowed and every girl's dance card had been marked by an eligible young man – precisely the sort of event Violet would have been groomed for had she not already succeeded in bagging herself a celebrated young surgeon.

Lily banged on the window of the bus.

Kitty mouthed, 'I'm coming!' and turned to Richard, smiling apologetically. 'Much as I'd love to, I promised I'd keep Lily company. I'd hate for her to be accosted by Dr Barrowmore from urinary medicine. He has terrible breath.' She giggled.

'Oh, you are a card!' he said. 'Well, off you go, I suppose! Can't blame a guy for trying, eh?' he said, winking. 'See you there.'

Kitty took her seat beside her friend, holding the wedding gift on her lap as though it was an unexploded incendiary bomb.

'He's still sweet on you,' Lily said. 'Richard, I mean.'

Kitty rolled her eyes. 'I know. But there's the slight problem of me not being sweet on him.'

Lily took out a salt beef sandwich and took a bite. She chewed thoughtfully then said, 'He's a doctor, though. If he'd asked *me* out, I'd—'

'You'd get bored within minutes, Lil. He only talks about himself. I can't be doing with a man like that, no matter how good a catch he might seem. My heart's just not in it.'

Lily squeezed Kitty's arm. 'I know where your heart *is*. I really can't believe you're coming to watch this.'

As the charabanc rumbled away Kitty raised her eyebrows and looked wistfully out of the window back at the Park Hospital clock tower. 'No. Me neither. I just didn't want to look like a bitter, washed-up old maid. Then she really *will* have won.'

The church was old, built in a pleasing reddish stone with terracotta-coloured mullioned windows. It took pride of place on top of a hill, from which branched streets full of grand Victorian and Edwardian gentlemen's residences. Now that the snow had cleared from their front gardens, Kitty could see daffodils, hastily trying to throw up their strappy leaves as if to make up for lost time. Buds on bare, gnarly cherry trees and tall rhododendrons showed promise of the spring colour that lay a month ahead.

She and Lily alighted from the charabanc.

'Crikey,' Kitty said, inhaling deeply of the sweet, unsullied air. 'Smell that! You can tell we're out in the sticks, here, can't you? I'll bet there's not a single house around here with an outdoor toilet.'

'It smells of pine trees!' Lily said. 'And money!' She laughed.

Kitty took in the affluent village scene with a city girl's tired eyes. 'Well, it certainly looks like Bowdon dodged the Luftwaffe.'

The grounds of the church were mainly flagged with old, flat gravestones marking the place where the great and the good of this small Cheshire parish had been laid to rest, many years earlier. Kitty thought it odd to be stepping over their remains, but there was no way to avoid them. The place was thronging with wedding guests – flamboyant women and dandies, all dressed in finery that certainly hadn't been run up in a damp Cheetham back parlour by an overtaxed seamstress with arthritic fingers. Surrounded by the wealthy and privileged who fleetingly cast a judgemental gaze over her and then hastily looked away, Kitty imagined poverty must be visibly clinging to her like the scum ring on an old tin bath.

'This is how the other half lives, eh?' Lily said, gawping at an impossibly glamorous woman's hat, which was a confection of petrol-coloured feathers.

Kitty grabbed her arm and led her through the rose-festooned archway into the church. Her thunderous heartbeat was out of time with the music of the church's organ. Through the mayhem of guests and family, she tried to glimpse James at the front.

'I don't want to sit too far forward,' she hissed into Lily's ear, grabbing her by the elbow. 'Honestly. I don't want to be seen. In fact, I don't want to be here.' She started to shake. 'I might just go.' The pungent smell of wood polish and winter roses was dizzying.

'Don't be daft!' Lily dragged her along a row, five pews from the back on the far right. 'We'll be fine, here. This is the wedding of the century. At least you can cheer yourself up with a damn good wedding breakfast at the end. I bet rationing won't affect *that*! I can't wait.'

Beyond the stone columns that propped up the vaulted, intricately carved roof, she spied James at last. He was standing by the altar, flanked by a best man whom Kitty didn't recognise but presumed to be the best friend he'd often talked about – Timothy, who'd studied medicine with him at Cambridge. The two men were exchanging words beyond Kitty's earshot.

James looked the most dapper she'd ever seen him, in a morning suit and pale-blue silk tie. His dark hair shone with Brylcreem, though there was no sign of a top hat. The sun streamed in through the spectacular stained-glass windows, dappling the floor where he stood with a rainbow of light. Yet James's face was pale and drawn. His conversation with his best man appeared to be grave.

'He looks nervous,' Lily said. 'Ha! I would be if I was facing a life sentence with Violet Jones.'

Kitty wanted to respond but found that tears were pooling in her eyes and her throat was constricted with grief. She shook her head and looked up to the ceiling, willing her body to absorb the tears.

'Are you quite all right?' Lily said. 'Shall we go back outside and get some air?'

Nodding in silence, Kitty left her wedding gift on the pew and followed her friend back through the hustle and bustle of the gathering congregation. Some were chatting with the vicar in the vestibule. Others were stationed by the exit, awaiting the wedding car.

Outside, the air now felt poisoned, rather than fresh.

'I think I'm having a funny turn,' Kitty said, clasping her hand to her chest. 'My fingertips are tingling. I'm woozy.'

'It's panic,' Lily said, leading her to a quiet spot where Kitty could lean against a stone buttress. 'We ought to go. If it's making you ill like this – There's being mature and taking the higher moral ground, and there's torturing yourself for nothing. Neither of them will thank you for it. They've both behaved like pigs. She bad-mouthed you, stole your man and then rubbed your nose in it. He let her.'

Kitty nodded. 'You're right.' She clasped Lily's hand and squeezed it affectionately. 'You've a wise head on you, Lil. But what I don't want is either of them thinking they've got to me. Does that make sense? I don't want to give them the satisfaction of knowing I'm hurting. Especially Violet. So, I've got to stay and get through this.'

She took a deep breath, stood tall and forced a smile onto her lips.

As they were about to go back inside, there was a rumble of a powerful car approaching, and a white Silver Ghost Rolls Royce glided into view. A pink ribbon had been tied from either side of the windscreen to the Spirit of Ecstasy silver figurine that bowed elegantly above the large radiator at the front.

'Oh, blimey. It's her,' Kitty said.

They slipped beneath the arch back into the church, peeping out at the scene where Violet's father was holding open the rear door, helping her to get out of the car.

Kitty saw acres of white silk, trimmed with mink and

a flash of red hair beneath a veil. The stragglers outside clapped when she emerged fully, like a dazzling butterfly escaping its cocoon and flapping its wings for the first time.

'I can't bear it,' Kitty said. 'Let's go and sit back down before I fall down.'

Several minutes later, when they were both installed in their chosen pew, the organist struck up the 'Wedding March' and everyone rose to their feet and turned to the back. Violet wafted into the church and along the aisle as though she were a Dior model in a Paris fashion show. She glanced from side to side as she went, beaming at her adoring public from beneath her gossamer-thin veil. The bouquet of white roses she held before her cascaded to the ground, almost grazing the trail of petals that her small blonde flower girl had scattered at her feet. Her veil stretched out behind her for several yards, carried by two red-headed bridesmaids, each of about eight years old and dressed in sugar-pink confections of taffeta and lace. Nieces, perhaps.

Violet's father linked her, looking regal in naval uniform, his jacket festooned with shining medals. At the front of the church, the vicar stood, smiling benignly. Violet's mother, the socialite, wore a smile so self-satisfied, Kitty was reminded of the proverbial grinning Cheshire cat that got the cream.

Kitty felt faint. There were only ten yards now between Violet and the grey-faced James. Ten became seven, became five, shrank to two – and there they both were. Ready to tie the knot.

Kitty swallowed painfully and held back a sob. She looked over at Richard Collins and berated herself for rejecting him, in part because she'd felt certain that James would eventually come to his senses and break off this charade of an engagement with Violet. Yet, here James was, getting further away from the possibility of a future with Kitty with every breath that passed through his body.

'Dearly beloved,' the Vicar began in a jolly voice. 'We are gathered here together in the sight of God . . .'

Kitty looked up to the ceiling of the church and silently prayed that God would send a miracle her way. None came.

The service moved along and presently, the vicar said, 'If any man can show just cause why they may not lawfully be joined together, let him speak now or forever hold his peace.'

Opening her mouth to speak, Kitty felt the truth trying to push its way out. She felt suddenly hot and started to tremble. Her face was numb. Her lips prickled. The moment passed, and the tense hush that had fallen over proceedings subsided, as the congregation exhaled in unison with relief.

Damn! Damn! Damn! Kitty bit the inside of her cheek until she drew blood, frustrated that she hadn't taken the opportunity to end this nonsense when she'd had the chance.

The vicar began the vows. Tears fell softly onto Kitty's cheeks.

'James Godfrey de Havilland Williams, will you have this woman to be your lawful wedded wife, to live together—?'

'Wait!' James said, loud enough to be heard from the back of the church. 'Stop!'

'James!' Violet said. 'Whatever is the matter, darling?' She turned to the Vicar. 'Please go on.'

'No,' James said. He took Violet's hands into his. 'Violet, I'm so sorry. I can't do this. I don't love you.'

'What on earth are you talking about? James! Don't be silly. It's just cold feet.' Violet's voice was shrill and full of fear.

James started to walk away from the altar and his would-be bride, retreating down the aisle.

'How could you do this to me?' Violet shouted after him, tugging her veil back over her head. Her face was a picture of immaculately groomed fury. 'Get back here, James Williams! Are you listening to me? Come back! Ooh! You absolute rotter!' She snatched her bouquet out of her bridesmaid's hands and hurled it down the aisle after him.

Her words went unheeded as James walked with haste and his head down towards the exit. Excitable chatter erupted in the pews as the congregation gasped at and opined about the dramatic jilting that was unfolding before their very eyes.

Meanwhile, Violet's father was hurling insults after the errant groom.

'You bastard, James Williams! I'll have you struck off for treating my daughter like this. You miserable, spineless – get back here at once!'

In the third row, Professor Baird-Murray lit a cigar and started to guffaw with laughter, his voice booming around the church, thanks to acoustics that amplified everything and made a mockery of secrets. 'Oh dear. Deary me. What a palaver. Jolly entertaining show, though!' he said, breathing out a billowing cloud of smoke.

The church was in uproar.

Kitty felt her cheeks flush hot as James neared the row where she was seated. She had half a mind to call out to him, but instead, she looked up at a stained-glass window that depicted Jesus on the cross and said a quiet word of thanks. She'd been granted her miracle, after all.

Chapter 42

The wedding guests drifted into the aisle of the church and descended on Violet, full of sympathy for the jilted bride. Yet Kitty could feel a frisson of excitement on the air as the upper echelons of Cheshire and Manchester society revelled in the scandal. This was what happened when your invitees were the glamorous and famous, Kitty supposed. Their concern was quite clearly superficial as they flung their arms around Violet in solidarity, yet left the church rolling their eyes and full of, '*Well I never!*' flabbergasted sentiment.

Breathless, she dragged Lily to the very back of the church, leaving the gift-wrapped fruit bowl on a table near the door.

'Do you think he's still here?' she said, emerging into the spring sunshine and peering down the street.

'Is his car here?' Lily asked, pointing to a row of rather grand cars that had been parked outside the local inn, across the road.

'I can't see it,' Kitty said, scanning the Bentleys and Jaguars for a simple Ford Anglia. 'But he must have been driven by his best man. I wonder where they were staying last night.'

She was desperate to find James and to question his decision. Had he been thinking of her when he'd walked away from his wedding vows, in front of some two hundred guests or more? Running into the street, she craned her neck to see if a lone man in a morning suit was visible in the distance.

Presently, the best man emerged from the church and lit a cigarette.

'Excuse me!' Kitty said, approaching him without a thought as to how it might look to Violet's friends and family. 'Are you Tim, James's friend from Cambridge?'

He nodded and exhaled a plume of smoke to the side. He looked like he'd just fled a pitch-fork-wielding horde of angry villagers. 'What of it?'

'I'm worried about James. I want to know where he went. I need to speak to him.'

Tim scrutinised her through narrowed eyes. 'Are you Kitty?'

She felt her cheeks redden to match her lips and coat. 'Why?'

'I'll take that as a yes, then.' He dragged on his cigarette. 'Look, James has got himself into a terrible pickle. I can't quite *believe* that he's just ditched such a beauty for . . .' The unfinished insult hung heavy in the air between them. 'You do need to talk to him, but perhaps give a fellow some breathing space for a while. That's my advice. Let him sort through this mess with Violet's family, first. There's a good girl.'

Kitty felt like a child who had just been told what to do by a patronising and not altogether well-meaning adult.

'You knew, didn't you? I saw you both talking at the altar,' Kitty said. 'Before Violet arrived. James looked like he had the weight of the world on his shoulders and he was telling you something.'

'It was just chat.'

'Why didn't you talk him out of it, if you knew he was having second thoughts? Why did you let it get this far? You're supposed to be his best man.'

'It was a good match.' Tim stubbed out his cigarette on the gravestone of a young woman who'd died long ago – the same age as Kitty, mourned by her parents. No children. No spouse. 'They'd been engaged for so long, it was starting to look farcical. And he told me there were family matters that were complicating things. You've clearly not met his father.'

'I know about his father. Look, I need to see him,' Kitty said, balling her fists. 'Where is he?'

'I can't tell you that, I'm afraid,' Tim said with finality.

As he looked Kitty in the eye, she noticed that his focus wavered. It landed on the inn opposite, before coming to rest on the redundant wedding car, where the liveried chauffeur was on his knees, pointlessly fastening tin cans to the bumper with long pieces of string.

'Please yourself,' Kitty said.

She found Lily queueing to get back on the charabanc to Davyhulme.

'I'm not coming back with you,' she said.

'But how will you get home?' Lily asked.

'Don't worry about me. I'll make my own way. I've got something I need to do.' She raised her eyebrows, silently communicating her plans to her friend.

'Are you sure?' Lily asked. She dropped her voice. 'Didn't you say something about not giving either of them the satisfaction?'

'That was then. When I thought it was all going to go ahead.'

'Well, if you're sure. Best of luck, chuck. And remember!' Lily stood on the first step of the bus with her impatient travel companions waiting behind her. 'Protect that soft old heart of yours!'

Without a thought as to how she'd get home on a Saturday, Kitty left the scene of high drama outside the church, where Violet was now in floods of tears, like a couturier's reimagining of Miss Haversham, and crossed the road to the inn.

Unable to stop grinning but knowing her endeavour could easily end in yet more disappointment and rejection, Kitty pushed open the door. She expected the place to reek of pipe and cigar smoke and to house a sullen gathering of scruffy men who had repaired there to moan about their womenfolk. In the inns that her father frequented, the men spent the afternoon supping soapy-looking ale until they were staggering around. This place was far nicer. The beamed, low ceilings and roaring open fires made it feel like an old farmhouse. Tasteful, rustic old furniture was scattered around in a sociable fashion. On a Saturday lunchtime, not long after opening hours, the place was empty but for a couple of well-heeled elderly gentlemen, sipping whisky by the fire with the remnants of a ploughman's lunch on two half-empty plates.

Where was James?

Behind the bar, the barman was smartly dressed in a shirt and tie, wearing an apron. The suggestion of a frown on his face said an unaccompanied, unmarried woman wasn't his usual sort of client.

'Can I get you anything, miss?' he said.

'No thanks,' Kitty said. 'I'm looking for a man who I think was staying here last night. A Dr Williams. He may have just come in. Dark hair. Dressed in a morning suit. Ring any bells?'

The barman shook his head but furtively glanced over at the door that led to a snug. 'Sorry. Nobody looking like that has been in.' He snatched up a tea-towel and started to wipe a pint glass.

She knew he was lying. Why was it that men closed ranks against women all the time?

'Thanks for your help,' she said, marching towards the snug door.

'Er, miss! I said he wasn't in here.'

Kitty ignored the barman, and by the time he'd lifted the flap of the bar to intercept her, she'd entered the snug. James was slumped in an armchair, staring dolefully into the flickering flames of a newly lit fire. There was a half-empty pint glass and an empty whisky tumbler on the table next to him.

'There you are,' she said, barely able to keep the delight out of her voice, though she knew it was entirely likely that he'd send her packing.

He turned around and blanched momentarily. 'Kitty!' His eyes were red-rimmed.

She could see he needed handling with care. 'May I?' She gestured to the chair on the other side of the small table.

He opened and closed his mouth as if the answer evaded him. She sat down anyway.

'I didn't think you'd come to the church,' he said.

'I was in two minds about it,' she said. 'Now, I'm damned glad I did. How are you feeling?' She was itching to lean forward and place her hand on top of his, but still wasn't certain if her presence was welcome.

James stared into the flames and raised his eyebrows. He puffed out a deep breath. 'Terribly, terribly guilty. Poor Violet.'

'Do you regret it – what you did?' For a moment, she was scared she'd misjudged his actions entirely. Maybe he *had* merely suffered from the proverbial cold feet and did still intend to marry Violet at a later date.

'You don't storm out of a wedding mid-vow in front of hundreds of people on a whim. I'd given it a good deal of thought. It's rather like I've been carrying a heavy burden on my shoulders these last couple of years.'

Their eyes met, and Kitty felt a jolt of energy course through her. She blushed.

'You look different,' he said, pointing to her lips. 'Like a film star.'

'It's just lipstick, James. It doesn't make me a better woman. I'm the same underneath. But you haven't answered my question. Do you regret walking away from Violet?'

He paused and blinked several times, as if considering his response. 'Absolutely not. I should have been man enough to reject her advances from the very start. She was never right for me. She met with my father's expectations, and that's no reason to marry in this day and age. Now, I'm free.'

'So, you just wanted to be free?' She could hear Lily's words of warning resounding in her head. *Protect that soft old heart of yours.*

'I wanted to be free of Violet. I wanted to be free of the sham of pretending I loved her when I knew I was in love with another.' He got out of his chair and sank to his knees before Kitty, taking her hands into his. 'The right woman for me has been there all along. I had her and I lost her through my own weakness and stupidity. Kitty, I love you with all of my heart and I always have. Can you ever forgive me?'

A wave of adoration for James washed over her, warming her to her very toes. Lily's words of warning were just a nagging whisper at the back of her mind. She was willing to risk all to be with the only man she had ever loved.

'Yes. Yes, I forgive you.'

James rose to his feet, pulled her out of her chair and took her into his arms. They kissed passionately, and it was as if the years of disappointment and loneliness were swept clean away. With her eyes squeezed tightly shut, Kitty could hear nothing but the hot blood rushing in her ears; she could see only bright lights like fireworks, exploding on the insides of her eyelids; she felt only the warm sunshine of absolute happiness, lighting up the dark, cold corners of the snug.

When they broke apart, James stroked her face gently. The skin around his mouth was pink with her lipstick. 'It's not going to be easy for us for a while. There'll be an atmosphere and tittle-tattle at work, of course. I can't guarantee Violet won't try to poison us both or engineer a nasty fall down the stairs! Then there's the small matter of my parents.'

'It'll be fine,' Kitty said. 'As long as you're not saying all this in the heat of the moment. As long as you mean it and it's not the whisky and chaser talking.' She looked pointedly at the glasses on the table.

His fingertips followed the curves of the demi-waves in her hair. 'This isn't the heat of the moment, though, is it? We've both had far too long to think about being together. Kitty, if you can forgive my past inconstant ways—'

'I already said I would.'

'If you can bear a man who works too much and sometimes seems withdrawn and who can't dance to save his life and who often misses the point of the joke, I'm all yours. I always was. If you'll have me, it would make me the luckiest man alive.'

They embraced and kissed again. Every fibre of Kitty's body seemed flooded with heady euphoria.

'Oh, and there's more good news,' he said as they came up for air.

'What?' She studied the deep laughter lines at the side of his mouth. 'How could anything match the turn this morning has taken?'

'Park Hospital has been chosen to become the very first National Health Service Hospital. We're going to make history, Kitty.'

PART III

—

1948

Chapter 43

'Now, Smith. I've arranged with Matron to nip out for a couple of hours, but while I'm away, I'd like you to give Mrs Bloom a bed bath. She's looking uncomfortable. Make sure those stitches are scrupulously clean and allowed to air dry.' Kitty studied the face of her new charge, Gertrude Smith. The girl was only nineteen, without a blemish, and looked far younger. My, how the junior nurses made her feel all of her twenty-seven years. 'Then I'd like you to help Bickerstaff to make up the empty beds for the new patients due on the ward this afternoon. Get you practising those hospital corners. There's room for improvement.'

Gertrude looked sullen. 'Yes, Nurse Longthorne.' There was no enthusiasm in her voice.

'And straighten your face, young lady,' Kitty said. 'Just be thankful you're not doing your training during the war. I learned my craft on dying men who had been shot to kingdom come. You think an old woman with weepy stitches after a hysterectomy is unsavoury, you should try treating a gangrenous leg stump.'

'Sorry, Nurse Longthorne. I didn't mean—'

'Now, on with the motley! I'll be back shortly.'

Making her way to the clinic where her father was receiving physiotherapy, Kitty descended the draughty stairs, looking out at the glorious early spring sunshine. How much the world could change inside a year, she mused. The previous March had brought the harshest winter on record to a close, ending with the demise of James's engagement to Violet; heralding the official start of his and Kitty's abiding love. The fortunes of the Longthorne family in general had improved in the last twelve months: Ned had finally been convinced to return to Manchester when four uneventful months in Liverpool had passed and still, his debtors hadn't taken what they were owed from his flesh. He had so far succeeded in keeping a low profile, navvying on the docks in Salford, albeit under the false name of Fergus Marshall, still living at home with their mother at her new Ordsall address. Kitty's father's spinal surgery had proven to be a partial success, at least saving his life, if not entirely guaranteeing that he could walk again.

As she entered the clinic, she found her mother shouting encouragement from the sidelines as the incorrigible old fool staggered away from his wheelchair, using a stick for support. The jacket sleeve that covered his arm-stump had been pinned behind his back, as was the case with many a wounded war hero. Kitty had no doubt he'd be spinning a yarn about his time in the trenches for any neighbour gullible enough to listen. Now, he was moving his feet with difficulty, but Kitty could see some improvement from his last session.

'That's right, Bert. You're doing lovely,' the physiotherapist said, nodding. She turned momentarily to Kitty's mother. 'Isn't he, Elsie? Just grand.' Her attentions returned to Kitty's father. 'Keep going, Albert.' She glanced up at Kitty. 'Oh, hello, love. Have you come to see your dad, taking on the world?'

'Blimey! He's like Jesse Owens,' Kitty said, chuckling. 'Are you going for gold, Dad?'

Her mother erupted into peals of laughter. 'Oh, Kitty! He'd give Hitler a run for his money.'

'Are you lot having a laugh at my expense?' Kitty's father said, his greasy hair falling into his eyes as his head shook with effort and indignation. He looked over his shoulder at Kitty and shot her a withering glance. 'I'd like to see you do this with one arm and gammy eyesight, to boot! I've got to wait 'til flaming July to get one of these new NHS appointments with an optician.' He started to lose his balance.

Kitty ran to her father's aid, as did the physiotherapist, and together, they caught him before he fell.

'Come on, you moaning Minnie,' Kitty said. 'Just you think about how things *could* have turned out for you.' She raised her eyebrows at him. Even as he neared fifty – an age when a person should have accumulated some wisdom and perspective on life – he was still as unappreciative as ever of the lucky breaks he'd enjoyed, including access to free ground-breaking spinal surgery, thanks to James's connections. Typical Dad.

Her father's thoughts were clearly on his criminal endeavours, however. 'I've only got myself to thank, me,' he said. 'Ingenuity. That's what I showed. I did my whack as a law-abiding citizen. When it came to the crunch, I did the right thing.'

'Give over, Bert,' her mother said. 'Let it lie.'

Kitty remembered the embarrassment of having to wheel her father into court, accompanied by her long-suffering mother, so that he could testify against his counterfeiting compatriots in return for dodging his own prison sentence. James had opted not to tell his father about that particular Longthorne family day out. 'I'm not talking about *that*, Dad,' she said. 'I'm talking about your operation. The fact that you're still with us, giving me earache and driving poor Mam up the wall. Statistically speaking, you should have died, and she definitely should have left you.'

Her father righted himself and poked at her leg with his stick. 'Some life this is! Having to be helped out to the carsey and have my arse wiped by my own wife.'

'Dad! Don't be crude.'

He gestured over towards Kitty's mother with his stick. '*She* does nowt but cock a snook at me, like I'm an idiot. Dog-dirt on the sole of her shoe.'

'Hey! Just you remember who cooks your dinner, Bert Longthorne!' she responded. 'One more unpleasant word out of you and I'll be putting Ex-Lax in your stew. You can get yourself onto the carsey. Learn to wipe with your left hand.'

He staggered three more paces, initially cowed by Kitty's mother's show of rebellion; then cheered by the physiotherapist's ensuing words of praise and Kitty's rapturous applause.

'Well done, Dad! You'll soon be hoofing it up the road to work on Shanks's pony. We'd better get you a proper job.' Kitty kissed him gingerly on his stubbled cheek and helped him back to his wheelchair, amid his constant grumbling.

As she hugged her mother and said her farewells to the physiotherapist for another week, she tried to swallow down her apprehension about her father's recovery. Kitty was not a betting woman, but she'd put money on it that her father would be back to his bad old tricks the moment he was able to walk unassisted. At the moment, he was under her mother's beady-eyed jurisdiction, and her mother had positively flourished since the power in their marriage had shifted to her. Who knew how quickly his mended ways would unravel, though, if he rediscovered his independence and the pub?

*

'Are you ready to go, Nurse Longthorne?' James asked.

Her beau was waiting for her in the foyer of the hospital, already wearing his coat and clutching his trilby. How handsome he looked today, yet Kitty would have to wait until they were in the privacy of his car before complimenting him.

'Yes. Thank you, Dr Williams.' She checked the time on her nurse's watch. 'We'd better make tracks if we're to make the train.'

Clutching her nurse's cape close against the fresh wind, Kitty accompanied James to his Ford Anglia. Wary of anybody watching them from the upper windows, they walked some distance apart as though they were nothing more than colleagues – a nurse accompanying a doctor to a professional engagement.

He opened the door for her and she climbed inside, barely able to suppress a grin, even after a year of their delicious, frustrating pretence.

'Wait until we're a way down the road,' he said, starting the engine and checking his mirrors.

They pulled away and, sure enough, Kitty could see Violet in one of the upper windows, watching the car and its occupants.

'She's still sore about it,' Kitty said, looking out of the back window and seeing her erstwhile friend grow smaller and smaller, finally vanishing from sight as they turned onto the main road, melding with the other traffic on the streets of Davyhulme. 'She suspects.'

'That's precisely why we're bothering with this ridiculous charade,' James said, smiling at her. 'The gossip behind my back is bad enough now, even when they think I'm a career-obsessed bachelor, with no time for women. Imagine how miserable our lives would be if we'd announced to the world that you and I are an item and have been since I left Violet standing at the altar?'

He indicated and pulled the car alongside the kerb.

'Whatever are you doing, Dr Williams?' Kitty asked coquettishly. She giggled.

'Being clandestine,' James said, leaving the engine idling as he leaned over and kissed her passionately. He placed his hand on her knee and started to kiss her neck.

She slapped him away playfully. 'Now, now! This is neither the time nor the place for a game of doctors and nurses.'

'Oh, darling,' he said, straightening up in the driver's seat. His cheeks were flushed. He took her hand and kissed it. 'Isn't it time, after a whole year, that we stopped this foolishness and went about things properly?' He looked deep into her eyes.

'You were just eulogising about how this "foolishness" has saved your reputation.'

'But I want you as more than my secret squeeze.'

Kitty sighed. She imagined James going down on one knee and proposing to her. She imagined having the wedding that had been denied to Violet and becoming a doctor's wife. She tried to picture the children they might have and the beautiful home they'd live in. 'If we marry, I'll have to leave nursing. It's unfair. I'm so close to being promoted to sister. And I love my work. You, of all people, should understand that.'

He nodded. 'Soon, though? We can't wait forever.'

'There's nothing to stop you proposing in the meantime.' Kitty raised an eyebrow. Her pulse quickened.

'You mean, you'd say yes?'

'Is that a proposal, James Williams?' She narrowed her eyes at him.

'I'm hardly going to propose to you in a car by the roadside, am I?'

With romance even thicker in the air than usual and Kitty left wondering if James was going to pop the question, sooner rather than later, they pulled up to the grand old building of Manchester's London Road Station. The clock high above them said the train they sought to meet was due to go in seventeen minutes.

'We'd better make it snappy,' James said, opening the boot and taking five parcels tied together in a bundle. He took Kitty's hand and pulled her through the hustle and bustle of travellers, carrying suitcases and trunks across the concourse to their desired platforms. Above them, letters and numbers rattled around on the giant departures board, as times and destinations changed with every minute that passed. Trains were heading everywhere to Newcastle, London, Birmingham, Scotland – all confusingly operated by two entirely separate companies.

The station was a noisy cauldron, bubbling with activity. Giant, shining engines stood on most platforms expelling billowing steam from their chimneys – some with a deafening honk of their horns. On one platform, a guard blew sharply on a whistle and there was a squeal of brakes as a train started to chug, chug, chug out of the station, giant pistons grinding away so that sparks flew.

They arrived on the platform for the London-bound train.

'Can you see them?' Kitty shouted above the din.

'Not yet,' James said.

'All aboard!' a guard yelled only feet away, giving a sharp toot on his whistle.

Thick smoke rolled in front of him from the braking train on the adjacent track, obscuring the view down the platform.

'Where are they?' Kitty said, panicking that they would miss their opportunity to say goodbye.

The smoke cleared, rising to the criss-cross vaulted roof of the station. There, only yards away, she spotted a crowd of about fifty children, holding the hands of work-worn mothers, clutching their cardboard cases. Some were in tears. In amongst them were five small, sorry-looking figures, looking quite lost.

'Quickly! Before they get on!' Kitty said.

They ran together down the platform and came to a halt before the band of unlikely travellers. Kitty recognised Dora Mackie's aunt immediately, clutching Dora's youngest in her arms. The old woman smiled benignly at her.

'You came,' she said. 'We wondered if you'd make it.'

Kitty threw her arms around her in an awkward embrace and kissed the Mackie children. They were dressed in their Sunday best. 'We wouldn't have missed it for the world.'

James crouched down to shake the hands of the three older children. 'Good to see you,' he said. 'I hope you're ready for the adventure of a lifetime. Have you made friends with these other young adventurers?' He nodded towards the other coughing, undernourished and delicate children who were also Alps-bound.

The small Mackies shook their heads.

'Ah. You will. You've got three months, cooped up together in a chalet with nothing to eat but delicious Swiss cheese and chocolate. Have you packed your skis?'

They started to giggle at him shyly.

'I say, Kitty. I don't think they've packed their skis.' He turned back to the children. 'I hope you've at least packed a nice warm pullover. Have you? It gets jolly chilly in those Alps, even in spring.'

The children looked questioningly at their aunt.

'They've got long johns and vests packed. They survived last winter, they can put up with a bit of snow. And if gets colder than that, I can always put newspaper under their togs,' she said. 'They'll be warm enough.'

'Ah, well, I've brought you all a little something,' he said, taking the bundle of individually wrapped packages from under his arm. He gave one gift to each of the children and passed the smallest package to the aunt for the baby.

The older children dropped their cases and tore open the wrapping with glee. They revealed beautiful cable-knit sweaters in the softest lambs' wool – shades of navy and blue for the boys, shades of pink for the girls. There were also thick-knitted knee socks and small shoe boxes containing sturdy brown leather children's boots.

'Clarks?' the aunt said, examining the baby's footwear gift. 'Fancy!'

'I knitted those jumpers and socks myself,' Kitty said.

'They're nice, miss,' the oldest lad said, rubbing the fabric between his fingers but still looking distinctly unimpressed.

After losing his parents to murder and the hangman's noose, Kitty was hardly surprised that the boy was unmoved. She felt a pang of sorrow in her heart for the children, wishing she and James could have done more for them than a three-month convalescent holiday in the Swiss Alps. She reached into her handbag and pulled out five large bars of Cadbury's chocolate. 'This is for the journey.' Ned's new job on the docks hadn't gone entirely to waste.

'Ooh, miss!' the children said, suddenly a good deal more excited. 'Ta!'

'All aboard!' the guard shouted again, blowing his whistle.

'Come on, you lot!' the aunt said. 'Get yourselves together or we'll miss the train.'

The crowd of youngsters clambered onto the train, supervised by several female teachers. Dora's aunt herded her little inherited brood on board behind them. Tiny, drawn faces and hands were pressed against the glass as the doors were slammed shut. Almost all were in tears at having to leave their parents and everything they knew behind, though the oldest among them may have been evacuated to places like St Anne's or the Lake District, during the war.

'Poor little blighters,' Kitty said, waving to Dora's orphans.

'It will do them a power of good,' James said, putting his arm around Kitty. 'Most of these children know little of the world beyond their street. Imagine what they'll make of mountains and forest. It was quite a battle to sort this out, but I'm glad I did. I can't think of anything better for a group of delicate children suffering from respiratory problems.'

'They'll love every minute,' Kitty said, wishing that Dora could have lived to accompany her own children on the trip.

The brakes were released and, with a jolt, the train started to pull away. Steam billowed onto the platform, drifting back from the engine, many carriages in front. Slowly but surely, the London-bound train snaked out of the station into the March sunshine, leaving Kitty, James and the still-waving mothers staring at the empty tracks, each wracked by a strange mixture of sadness and hope.

Chapter 44

'Get that bunting up, Schwartz,' Professor Baird-Murray told Lily, chewing on his unlit pipe. He pointed to a crate full of red, white and blue triangles that was sitting on the sister's desk in the ward. 'If we absolutely must be the first NHS hospital, I want that idiot Welshman, Nye Bevan, to know what calibre of hospital he's dealing with. This place has to be spick and span by tomorrow.'

'It's always spick and span, professor,' Lily said, pulling out the bunting that had last been hung during VE day celebrations.

Kitty put down the notes she had been reading and moved to Lily's side. 'Can't we find some men to do that, professor? We're terribly understaffed as it is, and I can't say many of us nurses are peachy about climbing up and down those rickety step-ladders.'

It seemed that everywhere Kitty had gone that morning, Professor Baird-Murray had been nosing around, barking orders to the nursing staff – though never to the trainee doctors – to tidy up, hang bunting, pin Union Jacks to the walls. For a man who had railed against the idea of a National Health Service for the past three years, now that Park Hospital had been chosen to be the first NHS hospital, with the grand opening ceremony to be attended by Aneurin Bevan himself, Professor Baird-Murray was treating the place as though it was his own house and he was hosting a wedding reception with King George VI himself in attendance.

'Now, now, Cecil, what's all this kerfuffle?' Matron said, barrelling into the sister's office, spotting Baird-Murray as he dragged the yards and yards of dusty bunting out of the crate.

Kitty grinned behind her hand. If Matron was calling the professor by his first name, she was clearly running out of patience.

'He's coming tomorrow!' the professor said. 'That bloody Welshman. We're going to be inundated by the world's journalists and photographers.' He grimaced. 'All scrutinising *my* hospital.'

'If it was good enough for Glenn Miller,' Matron said, 'it'll pass muster with the health minister.'

'We're not entertaining troops anymore, matron. They were easily pleased! Tomorrow, we'll be making history. Right now, you're working for Lancashire County Council. Tomorrow, you'll be a government employee. It's all change! And lily-livered quislings like Dr Williams can't wait to bow down to Bevan, the medical Führer.'

'Professor! There's no need for such churlishness. Not this late in the day. We have to accept change because it's knocking on our door, whether you want it or not. Now, stop worrying. They picked us because we're the newest and best hospital in Manchester. Much of that success is down to you, Cecil, because you've been here since God was a boy!'

He harrumphed with begrudging mirth.

'Now, stop haranguing my nursing staff,' she went on. 'If you want bunting hung, put yourself together an army of orderlies and off-duty ambulance drivers. My girls are busy, aren't you?'

'Run off our feet,' Kitty said, not appreciating the professor's implicit criticism of James that he was akin to the puppet politicians of Norway who had done the Nazi's bidding during the war. What a cantankerous old duffer he was! 'I've got three advanced cases of cancer, one stroke, two heart attacks and a bout of septicaemia on this ward alone. Come on, Schwartz. Let's leave the professor to it. I'm sure Mr Bevan will prefer to open a hospital where the patients are still alive.'

Kitty felt terribly daring for answering the professor back, but in truth, there was such an air of festivity and frivolity in the hospital with the impending grand opening, that she knew she could get away with some gentle joshing. Park Hospital was about to make history, and for a moment, rationing and poverty and the nation's dreadful post-war health shared a stage with optimism and hope for the future, all flatteringly lit in the July sunshine.

'We're having a rehearsal in the gardens in an hour,' the professor said, checking his watch. 'Don't be late, ladies!'

Rolling her eyes when her back was turned, Kitty allowed herself a satisfied smile. For all the senior consultants had railed against the idea of a National Health Service for years, here they were, preparing to open their doors to anybody who needed treatment, regardless of their ability to pay. No more need to steal penicillin if women like her mother suffered life-threatening infections. No need to rely on the charity of doctors like James, if Ned or his ilk needed more pioneering plastic surgery. No need for children like those of Dora Mackie to become dangerously ill before they might be seen by a doctor. Things were definitely on the up for everyone.

She looked out of the window and spied Violet below, bursting into gales of laughter as she shared some joke with a blushing Richard Collins.

Things were definitely on the up for Violet, it would seem. Now *that* was something to be thankful for!

Chapter 45

'Are you ready to meet your new boss?' Kitty asked James the following morning. They were poised to part company at the bottom of a staircase – he, repairing to the staffroom for a consultants' briefing over Bevan's visit; she, heading for the ward to relieve the nightshift nurses.

'Ready as I'll ever be,' James said. 'Out with the old and in with the new. Are you ready?'

Kitty nodded. 'Let's hope this new NHS brings some other changes for the better.'

She could see that James knew exactly what she meant. Kitty was hoping that the rules on nurses being able to marry and stay in the profession might become more flexible. Though James hadn't yet proposed, she didn't want to be forced to choose between the man she loved and the career she believed in.

James closed his eyes and breathed in deeply through his nose. He opened them again and smiled at her. 'You can smell progress on the air!'

Kitty laughed and slapped him playfully on the chest. 'Listen, you've fought hard for this, Dr Williams,' she said. 'Enjoy your big day with the big-wig.'

Throughout the hospital, there was a fizz of anticipation of what was to come. Bunting was now strung all around like colourful spiders' webs, brightening even the darkest corners of the hospital. Every nurse seemed to look even crisper than usual. Every doctor was wearing his very best suit, with his shoes polished even more highly than usual. Outside, in the grounds, the press were gathering, screwing long lenses onto bulky camera apparatus and checking their notebooks.

As she was about to enter the ward, Kitty overheard a terribly excitable Violet, who was walking briskly down the corridor with another nurse, chatting ten to the dozen.

'Oh, didn't I tell you? That dashing chap in the sheep-skin flying jacket asked to take my photo,' Violet told her companion. 'Turns out, he's only a photographer from a magazine! I'm sure he said he was putting together a feature about Britain's loveliest nurses.' She squealed with delighted. 'Do you think he'll put me on the cover?'

'Not half!' the other nurse said. 'The headline will be "Nursing's answer to Rita Hayworth"!'

The two scurried down the corridor in a fit of giggles, leaving Kitty to turn her thoughts to her patients. She entered the ward.

'How were things overnight?' she asked the night-shift nurse.

'Quiet, apart from Mrs Jenkins with her gallstones,' her compatriot said, rubbing the dark circles beneath her eyes and yawning. 'I can't wait to have a kip, except we've got Nye Bevan turning up soon. How am I supposed to get any rest with all that going on? Everyone's been told to line up in the gardens to greet him in a guard of honour. You'd think it was the second coming.'

Kitty chuckled. 'I doubt I'll even get to see him, knowing my luck. How's Miss Grimshaw with the septicaemia? Is she responding to the antibiotics?'

Her night-shift counterpart nodded and peered down the ward. 'Her colour's much better. Her blood pressure's fine. I'm waiting on her latest blood-test results. Honestly, though. Treating girls who've had backstreet abortions doesn't get any easier, does it?'

Shaking her head, Kitty thought about the risks she'd been taking with James when they'd had the opportunity to get away for a weekend together. 'There but for the grace of God go I,' she said. 'Women get a raw deal. Any new admissions?'

'No. But guess what? I heard that they've just had a girl come in with acute nephritis on Ward Five. Professor Baird-Murray says she's to be presented as the NHS's first official patient. There's a photographer going to be knocking around, later.'

'Oh, flipping heck,' Kitty said. 'I hope Bevan doesn't come in here. The last thing we need is the ward turning into a circus, and patients with serious ailments being treated as a curiosity. What's the girl's name? The one with the liver condition.'

'Sylvia Buckingham.'

'Poor lamb. You watch. She'll never live it down!'

Kitty scrubbed her hands and arms to the elbow and made her way down the ward to see her patient, Agnes Grimshaw, who was due a painful shot of penicillin. She stroked the girl's hair.

'How are you doing, lovey?'

Agnes smiled weakly at her. 'My mam'll be over the moon,' she said.

'How's that? Will she be pleased at the recovery you're making?' Kitty thought that Agnes's finely plucked eyebrows made her look far older than her sixteen years. With her bleached, wavy hair, she looked like a high-school Jean Harlow. But she was just another young girl, fed a pack of lies by some sweet-talking seducer and left holding the baby, with her romantic dreams shattered and her body in ruins.

'She'll just be chuffed she won't have to pay for her treatment, now.'

Glancing down the ward at the patients, who were a mix of those who had been able to afford to pay for private treatment and those who were poor and had relied on the charitable goodwill of consultants on admission, Kitty realised that the success of the NHS – the new great leveller – would depend on money. Money, or the lack of it, governed everything.

Kitty patted her charge's hand. 'Just thank your lucky stars you were born in a medical age,' she said, 'and that this happened at the start of the NHS. Do me a favour, love. Look after yourself better, when you're back on your feet. Don't give it away to every Tom, Dick and Harry.'

The girl started to weep silently. 'Who's going to look twice at me after this? My name's mud, and the doctor told me I can't have children if I get married. Not now. I wish I'd kept my baby!' Her silent weeping turned to heavy sobs.

Kitty put her arm around her and stroked her hair. 'There, there, Agnes. Let it out, lovey. That's right. You have a good cry.'

Outside, she could hear the commotion of everybody gathering for the health minister's visit.

'Nurse! Nurse! My bag's full and I'm uncomfy!' Across the way, another patient started to complain about her catheter.

'Nurse Schwartz!' Kitty said, trying to attract Lily's attention.

It was no use, though. Lily was tending to a woman who had just been brought up from theatre after heart surgery. Kitty searched the ward for the junior nurses, but they were in the middle of giving a patient a bed bath, as she'd instructed them to, and they hadn't yet been taught how to change a catheter. There was no way Kitty could just push Agnes away, however. There was still her penicillin to administer . . .

'Longthorne!' The ward door had swung open and Matron was standing by the entrance, calling her. She was red in the face and her eyes shone with excitement behind those glasses. 'Are you coming down? Schwartz! You too. It's time. He's here!'

Kitty shook her head. 'Sorry, matron. Things have just got – we're really busy. Enjoy your moment of glory. You deserve it!'

Though she knew nurses like Violet would love every minute of the press attention, Kitty was privately relieved that she was too busy to be a part of the grand opening madness. She didn't want to shake Aneurin Bevan's hand. What could she say to a man like that inside half a minute? She didn't want a photographer taking her photo. No. Kitty was happy to continue with her work.

Within fifteen minutes, she'd settled Agnes, had changed a catheter and had refreshed the dressing on Mrs Davies' ulcerated leg. Finally, she got a moment to peer out of the window at the scene below.

All of the available nurses had formed a guard of honour along either side of the wide path that divided the gardens, ushering Bevan towards the main entrance. Bevan himself was an imposing figure in a dark suit – his bushy eyebrows were visible even from where Kitty was standing. He was flanked by Professor Baird-Murray and Sir Basil Ryder-Smith and trailed by some other consultants from the board, including James. Kitty was so very tempted to wave to her beau, but, though they weren't far from her window now,

James wouldn't see her. Matron was the only woman in the company of dignitaries. She seemed to be leading the guided tour. How novel!

At the head of the group, photographers took photos of the momentous occasion. Bevan paused at the request of the journalists to have his photo taken. As the group milled about, Kitty could hear their conversation through the open window. Bevan was asking James about his ground-breaking work in the field of plastic surgery.

Kitty felt a warm glow spread across her chest as James answered.

'Of course, I couldn't have made such enormous gains in my field without excellent nursing support in theatre and recovery,' he said. 'The nursing staff at Park Hospital really is outstanding. And the best nurse I've ever worked with is so dedicated that I hear she can't even leave her charges on the ward to come and meet you.'

'Oh, really? That *is* dedication! What's her name?' Bevan spoke with a Welsh lilt to his voice.

'Her name's Kitty Longthorne.'

'Well, the NHS is lucky to have her. It's a shame to miss her,' Bevan said. 'We need more like Kitty.'

'Oh, there's not another gal like Kitty. She's one of a kind.' James smiled and looked at his shoes.

From her vantage point on the other side of the window, Kitty grinned. 'Daft ha'peth,' she said beneath her breath.

It was only as she started to shut the window that she realised a photographer was standing right next to her. He was a dashing-looking young man in a sheepskin flying jacket – the kind the men wore in the RAF.

'Sorry, nurse,' he said. 'I didn't mean to startle you. I was just getting a photo. The angle's better up here.'

He paused and studied her face. 'Can I take your picture? I'm doing a feature on nurses. I think you've got a good look.'

'Oh, I think you must have something in your eye, love,' Kitty said, clutching the bib of her apron tight.

'Please?'

Reluctantly, she posed next to old Mrs Davies who was absolutely loving the attention.

'Pretend you're taking her temperature!' the photographer suggested.

Kitty rolled her eyes and put a thermometer in Mrs Davies' mouth. 'Make it snappy. I've got patients to tend to.'

With a bright flash, despite her best intentions, Kitty was caught on camera.

'You're now immortalised in black and white,' the photographer said. 'Thanks. It's a great shot. In fact, if my hunch is correct, this will be the cover.'

It was only then that Kitty realised the feature she'd posed for – Britain's Loveliest Nurses. Already able to see the disbelief and envy in Violet's eyes, she glowed with embarrassment.

'Oh, you're joking. Don't be using that! There's a nurse called Violet. Red-head. Glamorous. She *really* wants to be your cover girl. Use her.'

The photographer shook his head. 'The camera never lies, miss. You're the cover girl.'

With the photographer gone and lunch being wheeled in from the kitchens, Kitty peeked again out of the window as she fastened a clean apron over her uniform. Outside, the grounds were peaceful once again, which could only mean one thing – Nye Bevan was on his guided tour of the hospital.

'Pray he doesn't come in here,' Kitty told Lily as they took the lids off the fish pie and carrots that were on the menu for the patients.

'They'll be down on Ward Five with that little girl. I don't think they'll bother with us.'

When the ward doors opened and Kitty saw a suited man in her peripheral vision, she froze. Clutching a plate in one hand and a spoon in the other so hard that they almost snapped in two, she sighed with relief when she realised it was James.

'Crikey, Dr Williams. I thought you were *him*,' she said, as he strode purposefully towards them. 'You nearly gave me a heart attack.'

'Well, you're in the right place,' Lily said, chuckling.

Kitty giggled.

James's expression was deadly serious, however. 'Do you have a moment, Longthorne?'

'Of course.' Kitty dished up a portion of fish pie and carrots, setting the plate and cutlery in front of a delighted-looking Mrs Davies. 'Fire away.'

'Er . . . in private.' James was standing with his hands behind his back. He was completely inscrutable.

'You'd better follow me,' Kitty said, leading him to an empty bed at the far end of the ward. If there were butterflies in her stomach, they felt more like wriggling caterpillars at that moment. 'This'll have to do.' She pulled the curtain around the bed and turned to James, dropping her voice to a whisper. 'Now are you going to tell me what's wrong? Aren't you supposed to have a clinic now?'

He was looking at her so intently that all sound on the ward seemed to still. She held her breath as he dropped down onto one knee. He took a small square box from the breast pocket of his jacket and opened it to reveal a shining diamond and opal ring.

Kitty gasped, feeling tears prick the backs of her eyes. 'Here? Now?' She was completely unaware of the sudden hubbub on the ward.

'I'm sorry it's taken this long,' he said, gazing up at her. 'But today seems to be a day for miracles and wonder, and I can't wait any longer. Kitty Longthorne, will you marry me?' James looked like a lost boy who was torn between fear and exuberant delight. There was no sign that he had heard the approaching footsteps either. 'Please say you will.'

Just as Kitty opened her mouth to respond, the curtain was swept aside.

'Nurse Longthorne!' Matron said, peering at them both with obvious surprise; the unmistakeable figure of Aneurin Bevan standing behind her. 'Dr Williams? What have we here?'

James scrambled to his feet, shoving the box hastily back into his pocket. 'I lost a cufflink.' Florid blotches of pink were already creeping up his neck and into his cheeks. 'Longthorne was—'

Kitty merely covered her mouth and stared at the health minister, lost for words.

'Never mind that,' Matron said, a glimmer of a wry smile tugging at her lips as she locked eyes with Kitty. 'I want Longthorne, here, to introduce Mr Bevan to the patients and to tell him all about what fine work we do on this ward.'

'Of course,' Kitty said, regaining her composure. She reminded herself to breathe; willed her pulse to slow. 'This way.'

Matron had already started to escort Bevan over to Mrs Davies, who was waving her pudding spoon at the health minister and shouting, 'Cooee!'

James slapped a hand over his forehead and sighed heavily. He muttered almost imperceptibly that he had to be in clinic, but Kitty grabbed his elbow before he could leave, knowing she only had moments before she was drawn into the fray around Mrs Davies' bed.

'Hey! Not so fast, buster!' she whispered. She narrowed her eyes at him but could barely stifle a grin. 'You don't half pick your moments.'

His dark eyebrows bunched together and the furrows in his brow deepened. 'I know. I'm so sorry. I didn't think—'

She placed her finger over his lips. 'Yes, James. My answer's yes.'

Epilogue

'How does it feel, then?' James asked, as they walked arm in arm in the early autumn sunshine along Sale's bank of the River Mersey.

Kitty came to a standstill and looked up into the canopy of blood-red leaves on a maple tree. Warm light streamed through the branches, kissing her cheeks. She breathed in the sweet air and held her hand aloft so that the facets of her engagement ring glittered in the sun.

'It feels incredible,' she said. 'All of it. Our engagement. My promotion.' She smiled widely at her fiancé. 'I think I'll insist that you call me *Sister* Kitty all the time, from now on. You doctors need teaching who's boss.'

'Cheek! Everyone knows I only answer to Matron.'

Kitty batted him playfully with her hat and chased him along the gurgling river until she was out of breath. When their pace slowed back to a gentle stroll, she looked again at her sparkling ring and reflected on the dazzling summer that 1948 had yielded. It was as though the sun had finally come out after a decade of winter.

Her father had started to walk again, albeit with difficulty. The glory of him needing a stick was that he was more likely to stay at home and behave than to abscond to the pub, where he'd almost certainly try to get embroiled in whatever scam was being brewed by the local bad boys. It didn't hurt that nobody would speak to him anymore, either.

Bert Longthorne had been labelled a grass. He would never be granted early release from that particular life sentence.

Kitty's mother had become the manageress in charge of the machinists at the raincoat factory in Cheetham. Her newfound responsibility seemed to have given her the boost in confidence she'd so desperately needed, and the decline of her husband's roguish ways was the icing on the slab cake. The two existed in a sort of entente cordiale in their Ordsall maisonette, and Kitty had finally realised that her mother needed to be needed, even if it was by a bad man. She'd known nothing but Bert Longthorne for all of her adult life. How could timid Elsie Longthorne countenance a life without her feckless husband? Being alone took courage, Kitty reflected.

'Better the devil you know,' she said aloud, watching the sunlight dance on the river's ripples.

'Eh?' James asked. 'Whatever's going on in that beautiful head of yours, Kitty?'

She leaned on his shoulder and sighed. 'I'm just thinking about Mam and Dad.' Her thoughts turned to James's parents. 'What a shambles our wedding's going to be. If a fight doesn't break out between your dad and mine, I'll eat my hat.'

James chuckled. 'I think we should run away and get married,' he said. 'Go somewhere romantic, like Paris or Venice and find someone to marry us there and then. Drag some old bat off the street to act as a witness and forget about our families.'

Kitty conjured a memory of meeting the Williams family. They'd met for afternoon tea at the Midland and had spent the entire time talking over her head about acquaintances from James's mother's bridge parties whom Kitty couldn't possibly have known. His father had talked endlessly about his days at Eton and Cambridge. He'd spouted on about the law and had reminded Kitty that her father was a convicted criminal. Everything that James William Senior had wanted to say about the Longthornes had been made clear in that one painful statement, made over a salmon sandwich.

'Running away is not a bad idea,' Kitty said. 'It's not going to be easy. Not if your dad's going to be such a –'

'Snob.'

Kitty nodded. 'And then there's Ned. They haven't even met Ned. By God. That's not going to be a barrel of laughs.'

The tendon in James's jaw flinched. He smiled, though it was more akin to a grimace. 'Ned's one of my success stories. We'll show my parents his face and tell them about his miraculous escape from a Japanese prisoner-of-war camp. If anyone can save the day and mend the bridges between the Williams and the Longthornes, it's Ned. Providing we ever see him again, that is.'

'He could be in the West Indies by now,' Kitty said. 'When that brute finally tracked him down and pulverised the new nose you'd given him, he said he was stowing away on a merchant ship, bound for the Virgin Islands or Jamaica. I should think he's on some beach, by now. He's probably married a local and has established a steady supply of rum to Britain at a gargantuan profit.' She chuckled, but the worry of her brother's incorrigible ways and the dangerous company he seemed to attract tied her stomach in knots.

'He'll be fine,' James said. 'I suspect he jumped on a train to London. He told me he had a girl down there. Ned's the most prodigious liar I've ever met, Kitty. And he could charm the girdle off Matron. He'll be right as rain. You mark my words. In fact, he's probably wooing Violet at the

Royal Infirmary as we speak, telling her his war stories and getting his nose fixed again.'

Pressing her lips together, trying and failing to keep the frown from her face, Kitty stopped and turned to James. 'Do you miss her? Violet, I mean?'

'Why would I miss her?' James said, kissing Kitty's hand. 'I'm relieved she's transferred. Don't you think the atmosphere's improved since she went?'

Kitty nodded. 'I don't think she will ever get over me being on the cover of that magazine instead of her!' She felt an involuntary mischievous grin spread across her face. 'At least Richard's followed her there. Last I heard, they were courting.'

'All's well that ends well, then, my love. We're to be married. We're going incredible places together in medicine.' He waved his arm in the direction of the warm yellow sun. 'The future's bright.'

'It is. It's a new dawn, all right. I feel like I've finally woken up from a long sleep full of nightmares.' She took James's hand and tightly interlaced her fingers with his.

'Rise and shine, Kitty Longthorne,' he said, kissing her gently on the knuckles. 'The storm has passed. The sky is blue. The world awaits you.'

Turning to face the city that lay in the distance, she nodded. 'I'm ready.'

Author's note

Dear Reader,

Thank you for taking this first journey through the late 1940s with Nurse Kitty Longthorne. Now that you've come to the end, I thought it might be useful to explain a couple of things about the story. I enjoyed writing it tremendously; in part, because it is based on some real-life historical events . . .

Though Kitty and her colleagues are all my fictitious babies, delivered safely onto the page by hands that were skilled in midwifery first, and writing, much, much later in my life, Park Hospital in Davyhulme really was the first NHS hospital in the country. Nowadays, it's known as Trafford General Hospital, and is a belting little place where I've been on many an occasion for all sorts of outpatient appointments. The staff is cracking (Hello to Paolo in Podiatry – he fixed my plantar fasciitis and got me back on my feet again with his excellent advice!). Back in 1929, however, it was opened as a cutting-edge hospital under the Poor Law, with 12 wards and 372 beds. Facilities included separate maternity, children's and isolation wards. It boasted up-to-date X-ray provision and even artificial sunlight! With its clean lines and simple design, you can really see the art deco influence in the main building and clock tower. Imagine how modern and smart it must have looked to the local residents who first used it.

Nurse Kitty comes to work there during the six-year period when the hospital was dedicated to treating the military sick and wounded – not just British soldiers but those from many other nations too. Towards the end of the Second World War, the patients were US airmen, but the hospital wasn't all doom and gloom. Concerts were held in the grounds to entertain the American troops, including performances from Glen Miller and the US Air Force Band. That must have provided hard-working nurses like Kitty with some much-needed levity, at a grim time in history.

When Labour swept to election victory just after the war, Park Hospital was chosen as the NHS's first hospital. After years of being pulverised by the Luftwaffe's bombs and suffering the effects of prolonged rationing, together with one of the worst winters on record, Manchester was more than ready for change. Happily, Health Minister, Aneurin Bevan ushered in a new, hopeful era on 5 July 1948. The NHS was born and Park Hospital made headlines! The hospital wasn't renamed until 1988.

I was a war baby, so I can just about remember the austere conditions, living in Manchester just after the war. We had very little and lived in a two-up, two-down with an outdoor toilet in the backyard. We used cut-up newspaper on a string, nailed to the wall, rather than toilet roll. Our only washing facility was the kitchen sink, where you could have a good strip wash. If you wanted a proper scrub, you had to go to the local baths. Nobody had a car until decades later. Nobody had a telephone. If it was cold, we slept with coats on the bed, and of course, it wasn't unusual in those days to sleep top-to-toe with several siblings in one bed. We ate a lot of potato hash, and you were lucky if you got corned beef in it. But I remember those suet puddings Mam made – jam roly-poly and custard was my favourite. She always said her meals would stick to your ribs, and by crikey, they did!

My mam and dad told me tales of their own wartime survival that left me wide-eyed, though never disbelieving. My mam was a machinist and my dad was in the catering corps, stationed in Wales for most of the war. Neither was educated or medical. To recreate the conditions of wartime nurses, therefore, I had to do a lot of extra research. Aside from interviewing retired nurses from that generation, the BBC has some wonderful online archives that supplied me with so much material for this book. Those women worked incredibly hard, cleaning, scrubbing, caring. The wards in those wartime hospitals were gleaming, cross-infection was rare, and nurses really got to know their patients during their stay. The hierarchy in hospitals was strictly adhered to, with the men being in charge, of course. Female doctors were a rarity, and doctors were treated like demi-gods. Matron, however, cut a formidable figure and was respected by doctors and nurses alike.

I've tried to give readers a flavour of a really good matron in this book – one who doesn't suffer fools gladly, makes sure the hospital keeps running like clockwork and who takes the pastoral care of her nursing staff seriously. Ultimately though, nurses like Kitty had to learn fast, work under pressure and do as they were told. They had little money, little freedom, and had to leave the profession if they married. It wasn't a career for the faint-hearted, but those women did a hard, hard job with enormous pride and care. I'm honoured to have told their story, albeit filtered through my own life experiences.

Finally, it's been really rewarding for me to tell readers a post-war story about Manchester. The city has a rich industrial heritage and a rich cultural heritage. There really is no other place in the UK like it, and I think it makes for an excellent setting for a saga like Kitty's. Crime and poverty are never far from anyone's front door, here; it rains for much of the year, which does my creaking joints no good at all! Yet the people are community-minded and friendly, always looking for the silver lining in those grey storm clouds and always willing to regale you with a funny tale. I hope, after reading this book, that you will grow to love the place as much as I do!

Thanks again for reading, and keep your eyes peeled for Kitty's next tale, where we'll see what the future holds for our brave young nurse . . .

Yours truly,
Maggie Campbell

Acknowledgements

Though my mother's and grandmothers' reminiscences about pre- and post-war Manchester are still vivid and detailed in my memory, writing about Kitty in the 1940s is a fascinating new adventure for me. I'd like to thank a few people who have helped me to give birth to this first book.

First, thanks to my agent, Caspian Dennis at Abner Stein, who is always happy to go down a road less travelled with me and see where it leads. He remains a steadying force, a professional rock and a true friend. He also has the best beard and owes me a jar of his home-made pickles.

Secondly, thanks to my editor, Sam Eades, who believed I could do this sort of tale justice. I hope you're right, Sam, and that *Nurse Kitty's Secret War* will be the start of great things. Thanks also to Katie Brown, who so thoughtfully edited the first draft of Kitty.

Thanks to the rest of the team at Abner Stein and the folks at Trapeze for their ongoing support during these strange COVID-19 lockdown times. To keep the British book-loving public entertained with the written word at such a dark hour, despite the logistic difficulties of publishing new books when the shops are shut and the world is stuck at home in pyjamas . . . that's no mean feat!

Many thanks to the wonderfully gifted and generous Gill Paul, who said such lovely things about Kitty! I'm honoured!

At the point of writing these acknowledgements, Kitty is not yet out in the world, but I'd like to thank the future readers and bloggers that get behind her story. I hope you enjoy reading the book as much as I enjoyed writing it.

Finally, thanks to my wonderful family for their continued support of my writing ambition.

Finally *finally*, I hope you'll join me in thanking the brave doctors, nurses and other medical and care staff who make the NHS even better than sliced bread! Not since its birth in 1948 has the need for our internationally admired and beloved NHS been so acute, as we battle on against a pandemic that has really tested the mettle of the nation, killing hundreds of thousands globally; sadly snuffing out frontline medical staff whose only wish was to save lives. I clap for them and I salute them all. Most importantly, I pay my taxes willingly so that they can continue the good work of keeping the nation healthy, regardless of status or wealth.

Credits

Trapeze would like to thank everyone at Orion who worked on the publication of *Nurse Kitty's Secret War*.

Agent
Caspian Dennis

Editor
Sam Eades

Copy-editor
Marian Reid

Proofreader
Laura Gerrard

Editorial Management
Sarah Fortune
Charlie Panayiotou
Jane Hughes
Alice Davis
Claire Boyle

Audio
Paul Stark
Amber Bates

Contracts
Anne Goddard
Paul Bulos
Jake Alderson

Design
Loulou Clark
Rachael Lancaster
Lucie Stericker
Joanna Ridley
Nick May
Clare Sivell
Helen Ewing

Finance
Jennifer Muchan
Jasdip Nandra
Rabale Mustafa
Elizabeth Beaumont
Sue Baker
Tom Costello

Marketing
Lucy Cameron

Production
Claire Keep
Fiona McIntosh

Publicity
Alex Layt

Sales
Laura Fletcher
Victoria Laws
Esther Waters
Lucy Brem
Frances Doyle
Ben Goddard
Georgina Cutler
Jack Hallam
Ellie Kyrke-Smith
Inês Figuiera
Barbara Ronan
Andrew Hally
Dominic Smith
Deborah Deyong
Lauren Buck
Maggy Park

Linda McGregor
Sinead White
Jemimah James
Rachel Jones
Jack Dennison
Nigel Andrews
Ian Williamson
Julia Benson
Declan Kyle
Robert Mackenzie
Imogen Clarke
Megan Smith
Charlotte Clay
Rebecca Cobbold

Operations
Jo Jacobs
Sharon Willis
Lisa Pryde

Rights
Susan Howe
Richard King
Krystyna Kujawinska
Jessica Purdue
Louise Henderson